CHRISTY M MOORE

Delicious Mediterranean Delights

Easy Recipes for Beginners to Embrace the Heart-Healthy Lifestyle

Contents

Introduction

Nourish your body, thrive in life. Embrace the Mediterranean eating pattern and allow your well-being to become your most valuable asset.

In the center of my bustling urban landscape, where the tempo of life moves at an exhilarating speed, I found myself at a critical juncture. The exhaustive hours spent in the workplace, frequent visits to fast food joints, and the burdensome stress had undeniably had a negative impact on my well-being. It was unquestionably time for a change, a change that would steer me towards the Mediterranean diet. Thus began my expedition, ignited by a cookbook that contained a plethora of enticing promises about a lifestyle that would benefit my heart and provide delectable dishes. Intrigued by the prospect, I made the decision to delve into this new way of eating. As a neophyte in the kitchen, the idea of embracing this novel culinary path was both intimidating and exhilarating. The first course I prepared was a Mediterranean salad. Crisp cucumbers, ripe tomatoes, and vibrant bell peppers gracefully adorned my plate, enlivened by the golden elixir of extra-virgin olive oil. The very first morsel I savored was a revelation—a burst of fresh flavors that reawakened my taste buds.

I felt invigorated, as if I had unearthed the sheer pleasure of consuming food. Weeks turned into months, and my culinary ventures expanded to new horizons. Roasted vegetables imbued with Mediterranean herbs quickly became a staple, alongside grilled fish and lean chicken. It was not a journey of deprivation, but rather an exploration of relishing genuine food in its most unadulterated form. As I continued on this expedition, I witnessed the transformative influence of the Mediterranean diet. My energy levels soared, and I began to shed the excess weight that had plagued me for countless years. My complexion radiated with newfound vitality, and my sleep became more restful than it had been in ages.

The Mediterranean way of life extended beyond just the types of food consumed; it encompassed a complete lifestyle. I wholeheartedly embraced the notion of leisurely dining, taking my time over meals, and fully appreciating every morsel. I found inner peace and tranquility in the process of cooking, as it became a meditative experience for me. Additionally, I cherished the social aspect of enjoying delicious meals with my loved ones.

During my annual health examination, there was a notable

revelation. It was evident that my cholesterol levels had decreased and my blood pressure had stabilized. Curious, my doctor wore a smile as he inquired, "What's your secret?" To which I simply responded,

"The Mediterranean diet." However, the true secret did not solely lie in the diet itself; it was the journey of self-discovery, nurturing both my body and soul, that made all the difference. It was a quest for equilibrium, a celebration of diverse flavors, and an intentional slowdown in a world that relentlessly races on. The Mediterranean diet has now become an integral part of my life, an emblem of well being and contentment. It has taught me that with a dash of culinary ingenuity and a whole lot of passion, we can transform our lives, one delectable bite at a time.

Why Choose the Mediterranean Diet

Opting for the Mediterranean Diet is a wise and health-conscious choice for various reasons. This dietary pattern is not only delectable but also renowned for its countless health advantages. Here's a comprehensive explanation of why embracing the Mediterranean Diet is highly recommended:

1. Heart Health: The Mediterranean Diet is widely celebrated for its ability to promote cardiovascular well-being. Extensive research has shown that this diet can effectively reduce the

risk of heart diseases. It achieves this through the inclusion of heart-healthy fats, especially monounsaturated fats sourced from olive oil, which aid in lowering bad cholesterol levels. Additionally, the diet encourages the consumption of fish, nuts, and whole grains, which are known to improve heart health.

2. Longevity: People residing in Mediterranean regions have some of the longest life expectancies worldwide. Their diet, consisting of fresh and minimally processed foods, is believed to be a significant contributor to their longevity. The abundant presence of fruits, vegetables, and legumes, along with a moderate intake of lean protein sources, has been linked to a reduced risk of chronic diseases, ultimately resulting in a longer and healthier life.

3. Weight Management: While the Mediterranean Diet is not a strict weight loss regimen, it supports healthy weight management due to its emphasis on nutrient-dense and low-calorie foods. The diet's balanced combination of carbohydrates, healthy fats, and proteins helps control hunger, and its focus on fresh produce ensures an adequate intake of vitamins and minerals without excessive calories.

4. Cancer Prevention: Research suggests that the Mediterranean Diet may play a role in reducing the risk of certain types of cancer. The high intake of antioxidants from fruits and vegetables, combined with the diet's anti-inflammatory properties, helps safeguard cells from damage and lowers the risk of developing cancer.

5. Improved Mental Health: Several studies have indicated that

following the Mediterranean Diet can positively impact mental health. The diet's components, especially omega-3 fatty acids from fish and healthy fats from olive oil, have been associated with a decreased risk of depression and other mood disorders.

Managing Diabetes: The Mediterranean Diet offers advantages for individuals with diabetes or those prone to developing the condition. This dietary approach promotes the intake of whole grains, legumes, and lean proteins, which have the potential to stabilize blood sugar levels. Additionally, the diet emphasizes the consumption of healthy fats, supporting insulin sensitivity.

Reducing Inflammation: Chronic inflammation is linked to various ailments, including heart disease, diabetes, and cancer. The Mediterranean Diet includes an abundance of anti-inflammatory foods like olive oil, fish, and a diverse range of fruits and vegetables. These components aid in diminishing inflammation within the body. Abundant in Antioxidants: Antioxidants shield the body against oxidative stress and damage triggered by free radicals. The Mediterranean Diet incorporates a plethora of naturally antioxidant-rich foods, such as fruits, vegetables, and nuts. Consequently, this diet helps prevent cellular damage and promotes overall well-being.

Sustainability: The Mediterranean Diet not only benefits personal health but also contributes to environmental sustainability. It encourages the consumption of locally sourced and seasonal foods, thus reducing the carbon footprint associated with long-distance transportation of goods.

Delicious and Ecologically-Friendly: Finally, the Mediterranean Diet is renowned for offering delectable and diverse flavors. It is a lifestyle-oriented diet rather than a restrictive one, making it more sustainable in the long run. By savoring flavorful dishes, individuals can feel satisfied while reaping numerous health benefits.

In conclusion, the Mediterranean Diet offers a multitude of health benefits, ranging from promoting heart health and longevity to supporting weight management, cancer prevention, and improved mental well-being. Making this dietary choice can contribute greatly to your overall health and well-being.

Chapter 1: Mediterranean Basics

Understanding the Mediterranean Diet

The Mediterranean Diet is a way of eating that draws inspiration from the traditional dietary habits of individuals residing in the Mediterranean region, specifically in countries like Greece, Italy, and Spain. It has gained recognition for its numerous health advantages and is widely regarded as one of the most beneficial diets worldwide. Let's delve into the fundamental components of the Mediterranean Diet.

Abundance of Fruits and Vegetables: The Mediterranean Diet places great emphasis on consuming generous amounts of fresh, local fruits and vegetables that are in season. These delectable foods not only provide essential nutrients, vitamins, and minerals but also supply the body with fiber and antioxidants that are vital for overall well-being.

Healthy Fats, Especially Olive Oil: Olive oil, a cornerstone of the Mediterranean Diet, plays a crucial role as a primary source of dietary fat. Enriched with monounsaturated fats, which are renowned for their heart-healthy properties, olive oil can assist in reducing levels of harmful cholesterol and mitigating the risk of heart disease.

Whole Grains: Unlike refined grains, the Mediterranean Diet encourages the consumption of whole grains such as whole wheat, brown rice, and barley. These varieties of grains are superior as they yield a higher amount of fiber and nutrients, thereby facilitating optimal digestion and providing sustained energy throughout the day.

Lean Protein: Moderation is key when it comes to consuming proteins within this diet. Lean sources of protein, including fish and poultry, are included in appropriate amounts. Fish, in particular, is a staple of the Mediterranean Diet as it contains omega-3 fatty acids, which are highly beneficial for maintaining heart health.

Legumes: Beans, lentils, and chickpeas are frequently consumed in Mediterranean cuisine and serve as excellent sources of both protein and fiber. These legumes are integral constituents of numerous Mediterranean dishes, imparting both taste and nutritional value.

Nuts and Seeds: Nuts, particularly almonds and walnuts, are often enjoyed as snacks or incorporated into various recipes within the Mediterranean Diet. These nuts are rich in healthy fats and protein, providing a delectable way to optimize one's nutrient intake.

Dairy products are incorporated into the Mediterranean diet in moderation, with a focus on yogurt and cheese. Greek yogurt is particularly popular due to its probiotic and protein content. Mediterranean cooking generously utilizes herbs and spices such as basil, oregano, and garlic. These flavorful additions enhance the taste of dishes without relying on excessive salt.

The consumption of red wine, in moderation, is a notable characteristic of the Mediterranean diet. Red wine contains antioxidants like resveratrol, which are believed to offer protection for the heart. However, it is crucial to note that excessive alcohol consumption can have adverse health effects. Therefore, moderation is of utmost importance.

Red meat is limited in the Mediterranean diet and when consumed, it is generally in smaller portions and often incorporated into mixed dishes.

In addition to following a healthy diet, maintaining an active lifestyle is a vital aspect of the Mediterranean way of life. Regular physical activity is encouraged to promote overall health and well-being.

Sharing meals with loved ones and friends holds great significance in Mediterranean cultures. This social element of dining fosters a sense of community and contributes to reduced stress levels, ultimately benefiting mental health.

The Mediterranean Pyramid

The Mediterranean Pyramid, also known as the Mediterranean Diet Pyramid, is a visual representation of the traditional eating patterns and lifestyle adopted by those residing in the Mediterranean region. Its primary purpose is to illustrate the core elements of the Mediterranean Diet and its related health benefits. In essence, the Mediterranean Pyramid is a modified version of the conventional food pyramid, with a specific focus on the foods and practices prevalent in Mediterranean countries. A detailed breakdown of the various components of the Mediterranean Pyramid, ranging from the foundation (foods to consume more of) to the apex (foods to consume less of), is provided below:

Foundation Layer (Physical Activity): At the base of the Mediterranean Pyramid lies an emphasis on regular physical activity and leading an active lifestyle, which are regarded as essential components of overall well-being.

Second Layer (Daily Foods): The importance of consuming a wide variety of fresh, seasonal fruits and vegetables on a regular basis is highlighted in this layer. These fruits and vegetables are abundant in essential vitamins, minerals, dietary fiber, and antioxidants that contribute to good health.

Third Layer (Weekly Foods): This layer focuses on the inclusion of whole grains such as whole wheat, oats, and barley in the diet, promoting their regular consumption. Additionally, legumes such as beans, lentils, and chickpeas are featured here as excellent sources of plant-based protein and dietary fiber.

Fourth Layer (Moderate Consumption): Olive Oil: Olive oil, especially extra virgin olive oil, is a primary source of dietary fat in the Mediterranean Diet. It is renowned for its monounsaturated fats and its ability to promote heart health. Dairy Products: It is recommended to consume yogurt and cheese in moderation as they provide essential calcium and probiotics. Fish and Poultry: Incorporating fish, like salmon and sardines, and lean poultry into your regular diet ensures a moderate intake of protein. Fifth Layer (Less Frequent): Sweets and Red Meat: Red meat and sweets are categorized at this level to indicate that they should be consumed less frequently and in smaller portions.

Sixth Layer (Occasional): Red Wine: Occasionally indulging in red wine is placed at the very top of the pyramid. This serves as a reminder to enjoy in moderation.

Top Layer (Lifestyle): Social Interaction and Enjoyment: The pinnacle of the pyramid highlights the Mediterranean lifestyle and the social aspect of eating. It emphasizes the importance of sharing meals with loved ones and friends as a holistic approach to well-being.

The Mediterranean Pyramid acts as a helpful guide to promote healthy eating habits and lifestyle choices that have been linked to a reduced risk of chronic diseases, particularly heart disease. It encourages the consumption of fresh, nutrient-dense foods while discouraging the intake of processed and unhealthy options. This dietary pattern is acclaimed for prioritizing quality over quantity and embracing the pleasure of food within the context of social interaction and physical activity. Ultimately, it contributes to a well-rounded and healthful lifestyle.

Stocking Your Mediterranean Pantry

Olive Oil Essentials

Olive oil plays a vital role in the Mediterranean Diet and is often referred to as "liquid gold" due to its numerous health benefits and culinary versatility. Below are some crucial aspects of olive oil:

Types of Olive Oil:

1. Extra Virgin Olive Oil (EVOO): EVOO is the finest quality and most flavorsome type of olive oil. It is made from pure, cold-pressed olives and does not undergo any refinement or chemical processing. EVOO possesses a rich, fruity taste and is abundant in monounsaturated fats, antioxidants, and phytonutrients

2. Virgin Olive Oil: Similar to EVOO, virgin olive oil is also cold-pressed and unrefined. However, it has a slightly lower quality and flavor profile compared to extra virgin olive oil

3. Pure Olive Oil: This variety of olive oil is a combination of refined olive oil and virgin olive oil. It generally has a lighter color and a milder flavor

4. Light Olive Oil: Contrary to popular belief, light olive oil does not contain fewer calories. It is actually a refined olive oil

with a mild flavor and lighter color. This type of oil is suitable for cooking at high temperatures.

Health Benefits:

1. Heart Health: Olive oil is particularly rich in monounsaturated fats, such as oleic acid, which are beneficial for heart health. It aids in reducing levels of bad cholesterol and lowers the risk of heart disease

2. Antioxidants: Extra virgin olive oil contains potent antioxidants like polyphenols, which protect cells from oxidative damage and inflammation

3. Anti-Inflammatory Properties: Olive oil possesses anti-inflammatory effects and may help mitigate the risk of chronic diseases associated with inflammation

4. Digestive Health: Olive oil aids in digestion and may alleviate symptoms related to conditions like acid reflux and gastritis.

Cooking and Culinary Uses: When it comes to cooking methods, extra virgin olive oil is most suitable for low to medium-heat techniques like sautéing, roasting, and pan-frying. It imparts a delightful richness to dishes. Salad Dressings: Olive oil plays a vital role as an ingredient in salad dressings, where its fruity and robust flavor can truly shine and elevate the taste.

Marinades: In the realm of marinades, extra virgin olive oil is often utilized to tenderize and infuse meats, poultry, and vegetables with its delightful flavor. Dipping and Drizzling: For those looking for an excellent choice for dipping crusty bread or drizzling over cooked dishes just before serving, extra virgin olive oil is a popular and versatile option.

Storage and Freshness:

Light and Air Sensitivity: It's crucial to note that olive oil is highly sensitive to both light and air as they can cause oxidation, resulting in a decrease in its overall quality. Thus, it is recommended to store it in a cool, dark place within a tightly sealed, opaque container.

Shelf Life: The shelf life of extra virgin olive oil is rather limited. It is typically at its best within one to two years from the harvest date. It would be beneficial to check the label for the "best by" or "harvest" date.

Quality: When purchasing olive oil, it is advisable to choose reputable brands that provide essential information on the label regarding the oil's source, extraction method, and quality grade.

Authenticity and Purity: To ensure that you are acquiring genuine olive oil, be vigilant for third-party certifications and seals of authenticity on the label, such as "PDO" (Protected Designation of Origin) or "PGI" (Protected Geographical Indication) for European oils. Caution with High Heat: While extra virgin olive oil is suitable for low to medium-heat cooking techniques, it may not be the optimal choice for deep frying due to its lower smoke point. When deep frying, it is recommended to use an oil with a higher smoke point, like vegetable oil. Olive oil is much more than just a flavorful and versatile cooking ingredient; it is also a crucial component of a heart-healthy diet. Its rich taste and numerous health benefits have made it a staple in Mediterranean cuisine as well as a favorite in culinary traditions worldwide.

Whole Grains and Legumes

Building a stockpile of whole grains and legumes is a clever and wholesome approach to ensure you always have nutritious and flexible ingredients available for preparing various meals. Here's a guide on obtaining and stocking up on these items:

1. Create a Shopping List: Begin by crafting a shopping list comprising the whole grains and legumes you wish to stock up on. Take into account your dietary preferences and the recipes you enjoy. Some common options include brown rice, quinoa, whole wheat pasta, lentils, chickpeas, black beans, and oats.

2. Prioritize Quality and Variety: When purchasing whole grains, prioritize items labeled as "whole" or "100% whole grain" to ensure they retain their nutritional value and haven't been excessively processed. For legumes, you can opt for canned varieties for convenience, but dried legumes tend to be more cost-effective. Although they require soaking and cooking, dried legumes offer greater versatility. It's recommended to choose a diverse range of grains and legumes to add variety to your diet.

3. Consider Bulk Shopping: Think about shopping in bulk to enjoy cost savings. Many grocery stores provide bulk sections where you can purchase grains and legumes by weight. Be sure to store your bulk purchases in airtight containers to maintain freshness at home.

4. Explore Online Shopping: If you prefer the convenience of

home delivery, you can also order whole grains and legumes online. Numerous online retailers offer a wide selection of these items, providing additional convenience and variety.

5. Focus on Proper Storage: Proper storage is vital for preserving the freshness of your whole grains and legumes. Keep them in a cool, dry place, shielded from direct sunlight. To safeguard your ingredients from pests and moisture, utilize airtight containers.

6. Labeling and Organization: To maintain the freshness of your food, it is advisable to label your containers with the date of purchase. Additionally, it is important to organize your pantry or storage area in a way that allows you to easily locate the grains and legumes you need for cooking.

7. Cooking and Preparation: It is worth noting that certain legumes, such as dried beans and lentils, require soaking and cooking before use. Therefore, it is essential to plan your meals and preparation accordingly. It is also important to keep in mind that different whole grains have varying cooking times. Therefore, it is recommended to follow the instructions on the packaging or research specific cooking times for the grains you have chosen.

8. Portion Control: When cooking grains and legumes, it may be beneficial to prepare extra portions and store them in meal-sized containers for future use. This approach not only saves time but also helps prevent food waste.

9. Explore Recipes: Once you have stocked up on whole

grains and legumes, it is exciting to explore various recipes that incorporate these ingredients into your meals. Whole grains can be utilized in salads, pilafs, soups, and as delicious side dishes. On the other hand, legumes can be added to stews, curries, salads, or used as meat alternatives in a variety of dishes.

By following these guidelines and adopting these practices, you can effortlessly build and maintain a well-stocked supply of whole grains and legumes. This ensures that you always have healthy and versatile ingredients at your disposal for cooking nutritious meals.

Fresh Herbs and Spices

Keeping a supply of fresh herbs and spices on hand is a fantastic way to elevate the flavors of your dishes and make your cooking more exhilarating and flavorful. Below are some guidelines on how to effectively stock and store fresh herbs and spices:

1. Selecting Fresh Herbs and Spices: Begin by choosing fresh herbs and spices that you personally enjoy and frequently use in your culinary creations. Commonly used fresh herbs include basil, cilantro, parsley, mint, and rosemary, while popular spices may include cinnamon, paprika, cumin, and oregano.

2. Opt for Fresh, High-Quality Ingredients: Whenever possible, opt for fresh herbs and whole spices rather than pre-ground alternatives. Look for items that are vibrant in color, emit a pleasing aroma, and show no signs of mold or wilting.

3. Plan Your Recipes: Prior to purchasing, take some time to plan out the recipes you intend to prepare and determine which herbs and spices they require. This will assist you in making the right ingredient choices and minimizing waste.

4. Visit the Farmers' Market or Grocery Store: Pay a visit to your local farmers' market or grocery store to obtain fresh herbs. Many markets offer a variety of herbs and spices in different quantities. For dried spices, explore the spice section of the store.

5. Storing Fresh Herbs: There are several methods for storing fresh herbs:

- Refrigerator Storage: Place the fresh herbs in a glass or jar filled with a small amount of water. Loosely cover them with a plastic bag and store them in the refrigerator. Remember to change the water every few days.

- Freezing: Another option is to freeze the herbs by either placing them in ice cube trays with a little water or packing them in oil. This preserves their flavor for future use.

6. Storing Whole Spices: Whole spices generally maintain their flavor and aroma better than pre-ground ones. Store them in airtight containers and keep them in a cool, dark place to ensure their freshness lasts.

7. Utilize a Spice Rack or Organizer: If you possess a multitude of dried spices, consider utilizing a spice rack or organizer to keep your collection well-organized and easily accessible.

8. Assign Labels to Containers: Affix labels to the containers or bags in which you store your spices, specifying the name and date of purchase. This practice aids in monitoring their freshness.

9. Grind Spices as Necessary: If you possess whole spices, pulverize them as required to maintain their potency. A spice grinder or mortar and pestle can prove invaluable for this purpose.

10. Dry Herbs for Future Usage: If you possess fresh herbs that you are unable to utilize immediately, contemplate drying them for long-term storage. Hang them upside down or employ a food dehydrator to thoroughly dry them before placing them in airtight containers.

11. Store Dried Spices in a Cool, Dim Location: Keep dried spices away from direct exposure to sunlight and excessive heat, as these factors can diminish their quality. A spice cabinet or drawer within your kitchen provides an ideal environment for their preservation.

12. Rotate and Replace: Regularly inspect your herbs and spices for freshness and aroma. Dried herbs and spices may gradually lose their potency, thus it is advisable to replace them when their fragrance diminishes.

By following these guidelines, you can ensure that your fresh herbs and spices remain at their best, enhancing the taste of your dishes and making your cooking experience even more delightful.

Chapter 2: Kitchen Tools and Techniques

Essential Kitchen Tools

Chef's Knife: A high-quality chef's knife is absolutely essential in my kitchen. It is my go-to tool for effortlessly chopping, dicing, and slicing all the fresh fruits and vegetables that form the foundation of the Mediterranean Diet.

Cutting Board: I always ensure that I have a reliable cutting board, preferably one that is easy to clean and spacious enough to handle the abundance of produce I utilize. Olive Oil Dispenser: It is incredibly convenient to have a dedicated olive oil dispenser or pourer at hand, especially when it comes to drizzling that exquisite extra virgin olive oil over salads, grilled vegetables, or using it as a base for cooking.

Garlic Press: Given that garlic plays a prominent role in many Mediterranean dishes, I heavily rely on my trusty garlic press to swiftly mince garlic without any hassle.

Mortar and Pestle: This versatile tool is perfect for grinding fresh herbs and spices, enhancing the flavors in Mediterranean recipes. I frequently utilize it to crush garlic with salt, create delightful pesto, or grind whole spices.

Citrus Juicer: I always keep a citrus juicer within reach to effortlessly extract the fresh juice from lemons and oranges, which is commonly used in dressings and marinades.

Baking Sheets: These indispensable tools are utilized for roasting vegetables and baking homemade whole-grain flatbreads. Their versatility makes them an absolute must-have in Mediterranean cooking.

Grill or Grill Pan: Grilled dishes are a significant component of Mediterranean cuisine; therefore, having access to a grill or grill pan is vital in order to achieve that perfect charred and smoky flavor.

Salad Spinner: My preferred tool for washing and drying fresh leafy greens and herbs is a salad spinner, which is a necessity when it comes to Mediterranean salads.

Non-Stick Skillet: When it comes to sautéing and cooking fish and lean meats with minimal oil, I opt for a non-stick skillet.

This promotes the healthy aspects of the Mediterranean Diet.

Saucepan and Stockpot: For simmering stews, soups, and preparing whole grains like brown rice, quinoa, and couscous, having a saucepan and stock pot is crucial.

Zester/Grater: To add zest to dishes by grating lemon or orange peel, a zester/grater is an essential tool. It effortlessly infuses citrus flavor into various recipes.

Food Processor: When making hummus, pesto, and other Mediterranean dips and spreads, I rely on my food processor.

Blender: Having a high-quality blender is vital for creating smooth and creamy soups, as well as making fruit smoothies and gazpacho.

Storage Containers: To keep fresh produce, grains, and pre-pared meals organized in the fridge and pantry, a variety of airtight storage containers is very convenient.

With these necessary kitchen tools, you can be able to effortlessly prepare a wide range of Mediterranean dishes that prioritize fresh, whole ingredients, vibrant flavors, and heart-healthy cooking techniques. This delightful combination ensures a delicious and health-conscious culinary experience.

Knives and Cutting Techniques

Mastering various cutting techniques and utilizing knives proficiently is essential for both efficient and safe food preparation. Below is a comprehensive guide on how to effectively use knives and employ different cutting techniques:

1. Grip and Safety: Prior to beginning any cutting task, it is crucial to establish a secure grip on the knife handle. Ensure that your hand is comfortably positioned and firmly grasping the handle, with your fingers securely wrapped around it. To maintain proper control, hold the blade between your thumb and forefinger. Additionally, it is important to always work in a clean, dry, and well-illuminated workspace. Avoid working in a damp or cluttered area, as it can increase the likelihood of accidents occurring.

2. Fundamental Cutting Techniques: a. Slicing: This method is ideal for achieving delicate and uniform slices of vegetables, fruits, and proteins.

> *- Begin by positioning the knife blade against the ingredient*
>
> *- Employ a gentle rocking motion, moving the knife blade up and down while maintaining contact between the tip and cutting board*
>
> *- Ensure a consistent thickness throughout the entire slicing procedure*
>
> *b. Dicing: Dicing entails creating small, evenly shaped cubes and is frequently employed for onions, peppers, and*

other recipe ingredients

- Commence with a sliced ingredient

- Gather the slices together and execute vertical cuts to form strips

- Rotate the strips by 90 degrees and proceed to make horizontal cuts, resulting in uniform cubes

c. Chopping: Chopping proves valuable for larger, irregular cuts, such as herbs and root vegetables

- Place the ingredient on the cutting board

- Perform a fluid up and down rocking motion with the knife, utilizing your free hand to guide the ingredient

d. Julienne: Julienne cuts involve producing thin, matchstick-like pieces

- Initiate with a rectangular-shaped ingredient and craft thin slices

- Stack the slices and lengthwise cut them into slender strips

e. Mincing: Mincing revolves around finely chopping ingredients such as garlic and herbs

- Position the ingredient on the cutting board and execute several horizontal slices

- Rotate the ingredient by 90 degrees and make vertical cuts, achieving finely minced pieces.

3. Choosing the Right Knife: Different knives serve different purposes. A chef's knife is versatile and can handle most tasks with excellence. For intricate work like peeling and trimming, a paring knife is the ideal choice. When it comes to slicing bread and delicate fruits, a serrated knife is perfect.

4. Keeping Your Knives Sharp and Maintained: Make sure to keep your knives sharp by regularly honing them using a honing steel. If needed, you can also sharpen them using a sharpening stone or seek the assistance of a professional service. After each use, hand washing your knives immediately and thoroughly drying them is essential to prevent rust. To ensure the safety of both the blades and your hands, store your knives in a knife block, magnetic strip, or blade guards.

5. Choosing the Right Cutting Board: It's important to use a cutting board that is gentle on knife edges. Opt for materials like wood or plastic, which won't dull your knife. Avoid using hard surfaces such as glass or stone.

6. Practice and Patience: Achieving mastery in knife skills requires practice and patience. Start by focusing on precision rather than speed, gradually increasing your pace as you gain confidence. Mastering knife skills and cutting techniques is a fulfilling journey in the culinary world. By consistently practicing these techniques, you will not only enhance your cooking abilities but also improve your safety and efficiency in the kitchen.

Mediterranean Cookware

The Mediterranean region is known for its diverse cuisine, and the cookware used in this culinary tradition reflects its rich heritage. Although there is no specific category of "Mediterranean" cookware, certain types of pots, pans, and cooking vessels are widely used due to their practicality and suitability for preparing dishes unique to this region. Let's explore some common types of cookware and how they are utilized in Mediterranean cuisine:

Tagine: A tagine is a cooking vessel made from clay or ceramic and is particularly popular in North African Mediterranean countries such as Morocco, Tunisia, and Algeria. This cookware is perfect for slow-cooking stews and braised dishes. Its unique conical lid helps circulate moisture, resulting in a dish that is moist and bursting with flavor. Tagines are commonly used to prepare dishes like Moroccan tagine with chicken, lamb, or vegetables.

Paella Pan: Traditionally used in Spain, the paella pan is a wide, shallow, and flat pan with gently sloping sides. Its design is specifically intended for making paella, a famous rice dish in Mediterranean cuisine. The wide surface area of the pan ensures that the rice cooks evenly, and it also allows the desirable "socarrat," the slightly crispy layer of rice at the bottom of the pan, to develop. The paella pan is essential for achieving the perfect paella.

Cazuela: Cazuelas are clay or terracotta cooking vessels that are utilized throughout the Mediterranean region, particularly in Spain. Available in various shapes and sizes, they are ideal for slow-cooking casseroles, stews, and baked dishes. Cazuelas are an excellent choice for preparing dishes like Spanish seafood paella or baked eggs with tomato sauce. The clay material retains heat well, ensuring even cooking and enhancing the flavors of the ingredients.

Olive Oil Decanter: Given the paramount importance of olive oil in Mediterranean cooking, it is common to have an olive oil decanter or dispenser in the kitchen. This tool allows you to effortlessly drizzle or measure olive oil when preparing various dishes. With an olive oil decanter, you can easily incorporate this essential ingredient into your Mediterranean cooking.

Couscoussier: A couscoussier serves as a specialized steamer pot exclusively designed to prepare couscous. This exceptional utensil consists of two pots: the lower pot for stewing vegetables and meats, and the perforated upper pot for steaming the couscous. The couscoussier is an indispensable tool when preparing delectable North African Mediterranean dishes, particularly the traditional couscous accompanied by flavorful vegetables and succulent meat.

Terracotta Bakeware: The Mediterranean culinary culture greatly appreciates the utilization of terracotta baking dishes and casseroles for various mouthwatering dishes. For instance, in Greece, these terracotta vessels are commonly employed when cooking moussaka, while in other Mediterranean regions, they are favored for baking delectable pasta dishes like pastitsio.

Grill: Grilling holds a fundamental position in Mediterranean cuisine as an essential cooking method. Therefore, it is not unusual for a charcoal or gas grill to be a prominent fixture in a Mediterranean kitchen. Grilled vegetables, meats, and seafood constitute staples in Mediterranean gastronomy, imparting delightful flavors to a myriad of dishes.

Tajine: Similar to its counterpart, the tagine, a tajine is a pot crafted from clay or ceramic materials, boasting a shallow, flat base and a lid. Traditionally, a tajine is primarily utilized for slow-cooking, simmering, and baking dishes prominent in Middle Eastern cuisine, such as the tantalizing tajine with baked eggs.

Olive Wood Utensils: Mediterranean cooking extensively makes use of olive wood utensils, including spatulas and spoons. These tools not only serve a functional purpose but also possess an aesthetically pleasing quality. Notably, olive wood utensils have the advantage of not affecting the flavors of the dishes, ensuring the preservation of the authentic tastes.

Copper Cookware: In certain Mediterranean regions, copper cookware, specifically copper pots and pans, enjoys significant popularity due to their exceptional heat distribution and control. This type of cookware is especially valued when preparing delicate sauces and desserts, as it provides an even and precise cooking experience.

In summary, Mediterranean cookware encompasses a range of practical and versatile tools that enable the preparation of dishes specific to this region's diverse culinary traditions. From tagines and paella pans to olive oil decanters, each cookware type plays a significant role in enhancing the flavors and textures characteristic of Mediterranean cuisine.

Cooking Methods

Grilling and Roasting

Grilling: Envision a passionate performance between cuisine and flame, where ingredients adorn themselves in the alluring attire of smokiness and fiery kisses. Grilling is a fervent tango, where open flames and meticulously prepared dishes elegantly intertwine. It is a mystical transformation that takes place when food encounters the fiery embrace of a grill. The sizzle and sear craft a vibrant mosaic of flavors, allowing meats, vegetables, and even fruits to attain a delectably caramelized perfection. Grilling transcends the mere act of cooking; it is an artistic expression, a primal connection to the elements, and a communal ritual that traverses beyond time and borders. It represents the embodiment of both simplicity and sophistication on a scorching hot, smoky grill grate.

Roasting: Roasting can be seen as the culinary equivalent of a cozy and thoughtful fireside conversation. It entails a gentle and patient union between food and heat, offering a delightful journey of flavors as ingredients luxuriate in a warm and enveloping oven. As food undergoes the process of gentle roasting, it experiences a remarkable metamorphosis, transitioning from its raw state into a glorious, golden, and aromatic masterpiece. Roasting is a remarkable fusion of scientific principles and sensory artistry. It exemplifies the meditative practice of coaxing out profound, earthy flavors, transforming humble vegetables and meats into luscious and succulent delights. The kitchen becomes a sanctuary of enticing aromas as ingredients surrender themselves to the slow and nurturing embrace of heat. Roasting extends beyond a mere cooking technique; it serves as a heartfelt culinary homage to the senses.

Sautéing and Stir-Frying

Sauteing: Envision a skilled chef in a bustling kitchen, holding a pan while surrounded by an array of fresh ingredients. Sauteing is the art of cooking with rapid, intense heat and skillful, swift movements. It is a passionate and dynamic dance between food and flame, where ingredients come alive with lively aromas as they spin in a pan. The sizzling and hissing sounds, the enticing fragrance, and the vibrant colors all come together as a symphony of sauteing. In this cooking method, small pieces of food, such as diced vegetables or thinly sliced meats, are quickly seared in a hot pan with a small amount of oil or butter. The outcome is a harmonious balance of tenderness and crispness, resulting in a delightful explosion of flavors. Sauteing showcases the epitome of culinary finesse, transforming raw ingredients into perfection within a matter of minutes.

Stir-Frying: Envision a bustling Asian street market, a sizzling wok, and a flurry of ingredients soaring through the air. Stir-frying is a lively, high-energy ballet within the culinary world. It is the art of cooking with speed and intensity, as vibrant vegetables, succulent meats, and aromatic sauces embrace the scorching embrace of a hot wok. The sizzling and popping sounds, the tantalizing aroma, and the whirlwind of colorful ingredients create an exhilarating sensory experience. In stir-frying, bite-sized pieces of food are tossed and tumbled in a wok, a wide and concave pan, over intense heat. The result is a joyous symphony of textures and flavors – crispy, tender, and bursting with the essence of each individual ingredient. Stir-frying embodies the essence of speed and precision, offering an adventurous and flavorful journey that celebrates the freshness and vitality of every bite.

Chapter 3: Breakfast Delights

Sunrise in the Mediterranean

Greek Yogurt Parfait

Crafting a Mediterranean-inspired morning meal with a Greek yogurt parfait is a delightful and wholesome approach to kickstart your day. Let's explore a straightforward recipe to assist you in this endeavor. Take note of the following ingredients:

- *1 cup of Greek yogurt (plain or flavored)*
- *1/2 cup of fresh assorted berries (such as strawberries, blueberries, and raspberries)*
- *1/4 cup of honey or pure maple syrup*
- *1/4 cup of granola*

- 1/4 cup of chopped nuts (like almonds or walnuts)
- 1 small ripe banana, sliced
- Optional fresh mint leaves for garnish
Now, let's dive into the instructions:

1. Preparing Your Ingredients:
Begin by washing the berries thoroughly and setting them aside. Slice the banana and gather the granola, nuts, and either honey or maple syrup.

2. Layering the Greek Yogurt:
To start assembling your parfait, place a layer of Greek yogurt at the base of a glass or bowl. Depending on your preference, you can opt for either plain Greek yogurt or a flavored variety.

3. Adding the Mixed Berries:
Next, generously sprinkle a portion of assorted fresh berries onto the yogurt layer. These berries not only provide a delicious touch but also offer a wealth of antioxidants and vitamins.

4. Drizzling with Honey or Maple Syrup:
To enhance the flavor profile, drizzle honey or pure maple syrup over the vibrant berries. This infusion of sweetness perfectly complements the tartness present in the yogurt and fruit.

5. Enhance the Taste: Generously sprinkle a layer of crunchy and slightly nutty granola on the top. This addition brings a pleasing texture and a subtle hint of nuttiness to your creation.

6. Include Sliced Banana: Adorn the granola layer with carefully placed slices of fresh banana. The natural sweetness and creamy texture of bananas complement the parfait perfectly, adding an extra dose of deliciousness.

7. Add Chopped Nuts on Top: Enhance the banana layer by sprinkling a handful of chopped nuts like almonds or walnuts over it. Not only do these nuts create a delightful crunch, but they also provide beneficial healthy fats.

8. Optional Layering: If the container permits, you have the option to repeat the layers. Begin with a layer of yogurt and end with a drizzle of honey or maple syrup for a touch of sweetness. This repeated layering adds depth and variety to your parfait.

9. Optional Mint Garnish: For a refreshing twist, consider garnishing your Greek yogurt parfait with a few vibrant fresh mint leaves. Not only do they add visual appeal, but they also contribute to the overall flavor profile, lending a subtle and invigorating taste.

10. Serve and Savor: Serve your Mediterranean-inspired Greek yogurt parfait immediately. To fully experience the harmonious blend of flavors and textures, make sure to use a long spoon that captures all the layers in each delectable bite. This visually pleasing and well-balanced breakfast is guaranteed to start your day on a delicious and healthy note.

A Wholesome Combination: Indulging in this Greek yogurt parfait is more than just a treat for the eyes. It offers a well-rounded nutritional profile, including protein from the yogurt, fiber from the berries, energy from the granola, and healthy fats from the nuts. Embrace the benefits of the Mediterranean Diet and relish this delightful creation as a nutritious way to kickstart your day.

Classic Frittata with Veggies

Crafting a timeless frittata enriched with vegetables is akin to conducting a symphony of vibrant hues and delightful flavors in the culinary realm. This remarkable masterpiece grants you the freedom to experiment with seasonal produce, resulting in a harmonious and gratifying dish. Here's an exceptional method to create a classic frittata:

Ingredients:
- 8 substantial eggs
- 1/4 cup of whole milk or cream
- 2 tablespoons of olive oil
- 1 finely chopped small onion
- 1 diced bell pepper (select your preferred color)
- 1 cup of halved cherry tomatoes
- 1 cup of fresh spinach or arugula
- 1/2 cup of crumbled feta cheese
- 1/4 cup of freshly chopped basil or parsley
- Salt and pepper to taste

Instructions:

1. Preheat the Broiler: Begin by preheating your broiler on the low setting. It will be utilized to cook the top of the frittata later.

2. Whisk the Eggs: In a mixing bowl, vigorously whisk together the eggs and milk or cream until thoroughly blended. Season the mixture with a pinch of salt and a sprinkle of freshly ground black pepper. Set this luscious egg amalgamation aside.

3. Sauté the Vegetables: Warm the olive oil in an ovenproof skillet, ideally a cast-iron one, over medium heat.
Add the finely chopped onion and sauté it until it turns translucent, which should take around 2-3 minutes.
Incorporate the diced bell pepper and continue cooking for an additional 3-4 minutes until it begins to soften.
Introduce the halved cherry tomatoes into the mix, and let them cook for another 2-3 minutes until they release their succulent juices.
Finally, add the fresh spinach or arugula, allowing it to wilt for approximately 1 minute.

4. Combine Eggs and Vegetables: Start by pouring the beaten egg mixture onto the sautéed vegetables in the skillet. Gently stir to ensure that the vegetables are evenly distributed throughout the eggs.

5. Sprinkle Cheese and Herbs: Next, evenly sprinkle crumbled feta cheese over the egg and vegetable mixture. For an added burst of freshness, sprinkle chopped basil or parsley on top.

6. Cook on the Stovetop: Allow the frittata to cook on the

stovetop for approximately 5-6 minutes over medium-low heat. The edges should begin to set, although the center will still be slightly runny.

7. Broil to Finish: Transfer the skillet to the preheat broiler, positioning it about 6 inches away from the heat source. Let the frittata cook under the broiler for 3-4 minutes, or until it becomes set and develops a slightly golden brown top.

8. Cool and Serve: Be cautious when removing the skillet from the broiler, as the handle will be hot. Allow the frittata to cool for a minute or two. As it cools, it will continue to firm up. Use a spatula to gently slide the frittata onto a serving platter.

9. Slice and Enjoy: Cut your classic frittata into wedges, similar to slicing a pizza, and serve it while it's still warm. The frittata is a masterpiece of flavors and colors, offering a delightful balance of textures.

This versatile dish can be enjoyed for breakfast, brunch, or even a light dinner. It's the perfect canvas for experimenting with your favorite vegetables and herbs, making it a unique and delightful addition to any Mediterranean-inspired menu.

Energizing Smoothie Creations

Berry Blast Breakfast Smoothie

Start your day off right with a Berry Blast Breakfast Smoothie packed with luscious fruity flavors and vital nutrients. Not only does this smoothie taste heavenly, but it also provides a nourishing and energy-boosting option to fuel your day. Here's a straightforward guide to preparing this invigorating beverage:

Ingredients:
- 1 cup of mixed berries (such as strawberries, blueberries, and raspberries) - 1 ripe banana
- 1/2 cup of Greek yogurt (plain or flavored)
- 1/2 cup of milk (dairy or dairy-free)
- 1 tablespoon of honey or pure maple syrup (optional, for an extra touch of sweetness)
- 1/2 cup of rolled oats
- 1 tablespoon of chia seeds (optional, for added fiber and omega-3 fatty acids)
- Ice cubes (optional, for a refreshing chill)

Step-by-Step Guide to Making a Refreshing Berry Smoothie
Follow these instructions to create a delicious and nutritious berry smoothie for a perfect start to your day:

1. Gather and Prepare Your Ingredients:
- Rinse the berries thoroughly, ensuring there are no stems or hulls remaining
- Peel a ripe banana and break it into smaller chunks to make blending easier.

2. Layer Your Ingredients:

- Begin by adding the mixed berries to your blender. If using frozen berries, set aside a few to garnish your smoothie later

3. Include the Banana:

- Drop the banana chunks into the blender, combining them with the mixed berries

4. Add Dairy and Sweeteners:

- Pour in the Greek yogurt and milk to provide a smooth and creamy texture to your smoothie

- For a sweeter taste, you can also incorporate honey or pure maple syrup at this stage

5. Enhance with Oats and Chia Seeds:

- Sprinkle rolled oats and chia seeds into the blender, adding a pleasing texture and a nutritious boost of fiber

6. Blend Until Smooth:

- Secure the blender lid and blend all the ingredients until achieving a creamy, velvety consistency

- For a chilled smoothie, consider adding a couple of ice cubes and blending them in as well

7. Taste and Adjust as Desired:

- Sample your smoothie and determine if additional sweetness is desired

- If you prefer a sweeter flavor, add a small amount of honey or syrup and blend again to incorporate

8. Serve and Enhance:

- Pour your Berry Blast Breakfast Smoothie into a glass, ready to be enjoyed

- If you saved some berries earlier, place them on top of the smoothie for an appealing visual touch

9. Indulge and Delight:

- Take a sip and savor the flavors of your homemade Berry

Blast Breakfast Smoothie
   - Enjoy its delightful taste while relishing the abundance of nutrients it provides
   Start your day on a healthy note with this refreshing and wholesome smoothie!

Avocado and Spinach Green Goddess

Crafting an exquisite Green Goddess salad with avocado and spinach is akin to summoning a lavish and lively garden onto your plate. It serves as a gastronomic tribute to the wonders of nature, where velvety avocado and tender spinach come together with a vibrant dressing infused with fragrant herbs. Here, we present a distinctive approach to creating this magnificent Green Goddess salad:

Ingredients:
   For the Green Goddess Dressing:
   - *1 ripe avocado, peeled and pit removed*
   - *1/2 cup of fresh spinach leaves*
   - *1/4 cup of fresh basil leaves*
   - *2-3 fresh mint leaves*
   - *2 cloves of garlic, finely minced*
   - *2 tablespoons of freshly squeezed lemon juice*
   - *2 tablespoons of plain Greek yogurt*
   - *2 tablespoons of extra-virgin olive oil*
   - *Salt and freshly ground black pepper, to taste*

For the Salad:
  - *4 cups of fresh spinach leaves, thoroughly washed and dried*
    - *1 cucumber, sliced into thin rounds*
    - *1/2 red onion, finely sliced*
    - *1 cup of cherry tomatoes, halved*
    - *1 ripe avocado, diced*
    - *1/4 cup of crumbled feta cheese (optional, for garnish)*
    - *Fresh basil leaves and sprigs, for garnish*

Instructions:

To create the Green Goddess Dressing, begin by blending the greens. Combine a ripe avocado, fresh spinach, basil, mint, minced garlic, and fresh lemon juice in either a blender or food processor. Blend these ingredients together until a smooth and vibrant green mixture is achieved.

Next, incorporate a delightful creaminess into the dressing by adding plain Greek yogurt to the green mixture. Blend again until all ingredients are well combined.

To enhance the texture of the dressing, slowly drizzle in extra-virgin olive oil while the blender is running on low. This process emulsifies the dressing, giving it a silky consistency.

Taste and make any necessary adjustments to the dressing. Add salt and freshly ground black pepper to your liking. If desired, you can also adjust the amount of lemon juice or olive oil to achieve your preferred level of acidity and richness.

To Prepare the Salad:

Arrange the Greens: In a spacious salad bowl, place the crisp spinach leaves as the lush base for your Green Goddess masterpiece.

Layer the Fresh Vegetables: Artfully position the sliced cucumber, finely sliced red onion, halved cherry tomatoes, and diced avocado atop the bed of spinach. This step introduces vibrant colors, satisfying crunch, and a delightful blend of flavors to your salad.

Dress in Style: Generously drizzle the Green Goddess dressing over the assembled salad, ensuring that every leaf, vegetable, and avocado piece is coated in this invigorating elixir.

Enhance with Feta and Herbs: To add an optional touch of creaminess and extra taste, crumble feta cheese on top. Complete the masterpiece with fresh basil leaves and sprigs as an exquisite garnish.

Serve and Relish: Present your Avocado and Spinach Green Goddess salad as an exquisite work of art, and indulge in the explosion of fresh, aromatic, and creamy flavors.

This salad celebrates the abundant green harvest of the Mediterranean and is certain to transport your taste buds to a lush paradise. It is more than just a salad; it is a delectable homage to the beauty and flavors of nature's abundance."

Chapter 4: Appetizers and Small Bites

Meze Magic

Homemade Hummus and Pita

Come join me in my kitchen as we embark on a delightful journey of preparing homemade hummus and pita bread from scratch. These beloved Middle Eastern dishes go beyond mere sustenance; they embody the essence of culinary artistry and tradition. Are you ready to immerse yourself in this flavorful experience? Let me guide you through the process with utmost detail and care.

Let's start with the ingredients for the scrumptious hummus:

- 1 can (15 oz) of chickpeas (garbanzo beans), drained and rinsed
   - 3 tablespoons of tahini (ground sesame paste)
   - 2 cloves of garlic, finely minced
   - 1/4 cup of fresh lemon juice (equivalent to about 2 lemons)
   - 3 tablespoons of extra-virgin olive oil
   - 1/2 teaspoon of ground cumin
   - Salt and freshly ground black pepper, to your taste
   - 2-3 tablespoons of water (adjust according to your desired consistency)
   - Paprika and olive oil, for garnishing

Now, let's dive into preparing delectable pita bread with the following ingredients:
   - 2 cups of all-purpose flour
   - 1 teaspoon of salt
   - 1 teaspoon of sugar
   - 2 1/4 teaspoons of active dry yeast
   - 1 cup of warm water
   - 1 tablespoon of olive oil (plus extra for brushing)
   - Sesame seeds (optional), for garnishing

Preparing the Hummus:

Blend the Enchantment: With the assistance of a food processor, merge together chickpeas, tahini, minced garlic, fresh lemon juice, olive oil, ground cumin, salt, and black pepper. Secure the lid with a whisper of anticipation.

A Swift Whirl of Metamorphosis: Process the elements until they metamorphose into a smooth, luxurious fusion. Witness the mesmerizing swirl of flavors and aromas dancing harmoniously.

Adjusting the Texture: Should the hummus prove too thick, gradually introduce water while blending until it achieves the desired consistency. Patience is key; allow the textures to blend harmoniously.

Taste and Refine: Savor your creation. Does it possess the perfect balance of rich tahini, tangy lemon, and fragrant garlic? If necessary, fine-tune the seasoning and bask in the sensory symphony.

Presenting the Artistry: Delicately scoop your homemade hummus into a shallow dish. Drizzle with olive oil and sprinkle a dash of paprika. The presentation serves as your artistic canvas.

Creating the Pita Bread:

Activate the Yeast: Combine warm water and sugar in a bowl. Sprinkle active dry yeast onto the surface and observe as it comes alive, producing a frothy and yeasty aroma. Allow it to rest for approximately 5-10 minutes.

Blend the Essentials: In a separate bowl, mix all-purpose flour and salt together. Add olive oil to the yeast mixture and pour this liquid elixir into the dry ingredients. The enchanting ritual commences.

Knead and Mold: On a floured surface, knead the dough until it becomes smooth and elastic. This tactile connection with the dough is where the magic occurs.

Rising to the Occasion: Place the dough in a lightly greased bowl, cover it, and allow it to rise until it doubles in size, typically taking around 1-1.5 hours. It is a patient and serene transformation.

Divide and Shape: Divide the dough into small and equal portions. Shape each portion into a ball and gently flatten them into circular shapes resembling pitas.

Heat and Transform: Preheat your oven to 475°F (245°C) with a baking stone or an inverted baking sheet inside. The intense heat becomes the catalyst for the perfect pita.

Bake the Bread: One by one, place the pita circles onto the hot baking stone. Observe as they inflate and catch their breath. It only takes around 3-4 minutes for them to develop a beautiful golden hue.

Embrace the Sizzle: As the pitas emerge from the oven, listen to their gentle sizzle. They will puff up and crack open, revealing their warm and fluffy interiors. Brush them with olive oil and sprinkle sesame seeds for an extra burst of delight.

The Grand Unveiling: Now, place your homemade hummus and warm pita bread side by side. Experience the marriage of flavors, the heritage, and the love infused in every bite. Enjoy the journey, as this culinary adventure is just as much about the process as it is about the taste. Bon appétit!

Stuffed Grape Leaves (Dolmades)

Creating stuffed grape leaves, also known as Dolmades, is an exquisite culinary adventure that seamlessly combines diverse flavors, textures, and cultural traditions. This delightful dish originates from the rich cuisines of the Mediterranean and Middle Eastern regions, encouraging you to immerse yourself in the art of meticulous wrapping and filling. Join me on this extraordinary gastronomic journey as I provide you with expert guidance.

Ingredients for the Filling:

- 1 cup of uncooked short-grain rice
- 1/2 pound of ground lamb or beef (optional, for those seeking a meaty variation)
- Finely chopped onion (1 onion)
- Minced garlic (2 cloves)
- Chopped fresh mint (1/4 cup)
- Chopped fresh dill (1/4 cup)
- Chopped fresh parsley (1/4 cup)
- Optional addition of pine nuts (1/4 cup)
- 2 tablespoons of extra-virgin olive oil
- Salt and freshly ground black pepper to enhance the taste

For the Grape Leaves:

- 1 jar of grape leaves preserved in brine (approximately 60 leaves required)
- Hot water for rinsing the grape leaves and removing excess brine

Cooking Instructions:

- Squeeze the juice of 2-3 lemons
- Incorporate 1/4 cup of extra-virgin olive oil
- Utilize either 2-3 cups of chicken or vegetable broth to cook the grape leaves thoroughly

Instructions:

Preparing the Filling: Start by sautéing the aromatics. In a spacious frying pan, heat up the olive oil over medium heat. Add the finely diced onion and minced garlic. Sauté them until they become translucent and release their delightful fragrance.

Adding the Protein (Optional): If you prefer a meaty version, you can include ground lamb or beef to the pan. Cook it until it turns brown and crumbles into small pieces.

Combining the Herbs and Rice: In a large bowl for mixing, bring together the uncooked rice, finely chopped mint, dill, parsley, and optionally pine nuts.

Incorporating the Sautéed Aromatics: Gently fold in the sautéed onions and garlic, along with the cooked meat if you choose to include it. This aromatic blend of herbs and sautéed ingredients will form the centerpiece of your Dolmades.

Preparing the Grape Leaves:

Wash and Soak: Gently remove grape leaves from the jar and rinse them under hot water to eliminate any excess brine. Allow the leaves to drain and separate them.

Wrapping the Dolmades:

Commence Wrapping: Place a single grape leaf on a clean surface, ensuring that the shiny side is facing down. Trim the stem and spoon approximately a tablespoon of the filling mixture onto the center of the leaf.

Fold and Tuck: Begin by folding the sides of the leaf over the filling. Then, starting from the bottom, roll it into a tightly wrapped, cigar-shaped bundle.

Seal the Bundle: Position the Dolma with the seam-side facing down in a deep, ovenproof pot. Continue wrapping until all the filling has been used.

Cooking the Dolmades:

Prepare for Simmering: Whisk together the lemon juice and olive oil in a bowl. Pour this mixture over the Dolmades in the pot.

Layer and Simmer: Carefully layer the Dolmades in the pot. Pour enough chicken or vegetable broth over them, ensuring they are almost covered. Place an inverted heatproof plate on top to prevent movement.

Simmer and Absorb: Cover the pot and simmer over low heat for approximately 45-60 minutes, or until the rice is cooked and the Dolmades have absorbed all the flavors.

The Grand Unveiling: Uncover your pot and savor the delightful aroma of herbs and citrus. Dolmades are best enjoyed when warm, often accompanied by a dollop of yogurt or a squeeze of lemon.

With each bite, you embark on a culinary journey filled with tradition and intricate flavors. Share your creations with loved ones and allow the Dolmades to transport them to the heart of Mediterranean cuisine. Bon appétit!

Mediterranean Tapas

Spicy Red Pepper and Walnut Spread

Introducing the Spicy Red Pepper and Walnut Spread: A Fiery Harmony Let's embark on a thrilling journey into the captivating realm of the Spicy Red Pepper and Walnut Spread, a lively dip from the Mediterranean that tantalizes your taste buds with a sensational blend of heat and nuttiness. This remarkable variation adds a unique touch to the well-known Muhammara recipe, renowned for its harmonious flavors and incredible versatility. Now, let's delve into the art of crafting this culinary masterpiece:

Ingredients:

- 2 sizeable red bell peppers
- 1 cup of toasted walnuts
- 2-3 minced garlic cloves
- 1-2 red chili peppers (adjust quantity to achieve desired spiciness)
- 2 tablespoons of pomegranate molasses (or lemon juice as an alternative)
- 1 tablespoon of ground cumin
- 1/4 cup of extra-virgin olive oil
- Salt and freshly ground black pepper, according to taste
- Fresh parsley, for an elegant garnish

Instructions:

Roasting the Red Peppers:
Prepare the Grill or Broiler: Start by preheating your grill or broiler on high heat. Our goal is to achieve the perfect charring of the red peppers.

Char the Peppers: Take the red bell peppers and place them directly over the flames on the grill or under the broiler. Allow them to blister and blacken, turning them occasionally to ensure an even char. This process is a delightful combination of fire and flavor.

Sweat and Peel: Once the peppers are evenly charred and their skin starts to blister, carefully remove them from the heat and transfer them into a bowl. Cover the bowl with plastic wrap and let the peppers "sweat" for approximately 15 minutes. This sweating technique makes peeling the peppers much easier.

Peel and Seed: After the sweating phase, gently peel off the charred skin from the red peppers. Cut them open, discard the seeds, and proceed to slice them into thin strips. Witness the incredible transformation of the peppers into smoky and tender delights.

Creating the Spread:

Begin by blending the base ingredients together. Using a food processor, combine the toasted walnuts, minced garlic, and red chili peppers. Pulse them until their consistency becomes coarse.

Incorporate the Red Peppers:
   Next, introduce the roasted red peppers into the walnut mixture. Pulse again, ensuring that the peppers are finely chopped and fully integrated into the blend.

Enhance the Flavor Profile:
   To add depth and zest to your fiery red mixture, include either pomegranate molasses or lemon juice, depending on your preference. Also, incorporate ground cumin and extra-virgin olive oil. These components will contribute flavor layers to the spread.

Achieve Balance:

Season the creation with a suitable amount of salt and freshly ground black pepper. Taste the spread and, if necessary, adjust the seasoning accordingly to achieve a harmonious balance of flavors.

Achieve Perfection:

Blend the entire mixture in the food processor until it reaches a velvety consistency and a beautiful, rustic texture. This step is crucial to ensure your creation is perfectly blended.

Enhancing and Relishing:

Present with Elegance: Transfer your Spicy Red Pepper and Walnut Spread into an exquisite serving dish. Add a touch of lavishness by drizzling a small amount of extra virgin olive oil on top.

A Hint of Freshness: Sprinkle the spread with freshly chopped parsley, creating a vibrant garnish that brings a refreshing contrast to the intense flavors.

Serve and Enjoy: Pair your Spicy Red Pepper and Walnut Spread with warm pita bread, crisp vegetables, or use it as a condiment for grilled meats. Observe as your guests delight in every spicy and nutty morsel. This spread is more than just a dip; it offers a culinary journey that exalts the bold and fiery essence of Mediterranean cuisine.

Share it with loved ones, allowing the zesty red peppers and toasted walnuts to ignite a symphony of flavors in each bite.

Bon appétit!

Mediterranean Quinoa Salad

Crafting a Mediterranean Quinoa Salad is akin to embarking on a delightful sojourn amidst the sun-drenched essence of the Mediterranean region. Allow me to share my personal method of concocting this vibrant and nourishing dish. The following are the ingredients I utilize:

- *1 cup of quinoa*
  - *2 cups of water or vegetable broth*
  - *1 cup of halved cherry tomatoes*
  - *1 diced cucumber*
  - *1/2 finely chopped red onion*
  - *1/2 cup of pitted and sliced Kalamata olives*
  - *1/2 cup of crumbled feta cheese*
  - *1/4 cup of freshly chopped parsley*
  - *1/4 cup of freshly chopped mint*
  - *Juice from 1-2 lemons*
  - *3 tablespoons of extra-virgin olive oil*
  - *Salt and freshly ground black pepper, to taste*

Now, allow me to guide you through the preparation process:

Cooking the Quinoa:
   To commence, I commence by rinsing the quinoa under cold water, thus eliminating any remnants of bitterness. Then, I

combine the quinoa with water or vegetable broth, bringing it to a vigorous boil. Once boiling, I reduce the heat, cover the saucepan, and allow it to gently simmer for approximately 15 minutes or until the liquid is fully absorbed and the quinoa attains a fluffy texture. Subsequently, I remove it from the heat, employ a fork to fluff it up, and let it cool at a leisurely pace.

Preparing the Vegetables:

As the quinoa cools, I proceed to prepare the fresh ingredients. I commence by halving the cherry tomatoes, dicing the cucumber, finely chopping the red onion, and meticulously pitting and slicing the Kalamata olives. The resulting assortment of vibrant colors and tantalizing textures is what truly makes this salad irresistibly captivating.

Combining the Ingredients:

Within a generously sized salad bowl, I artfully combine the cooked quinoa, cherry tomatoes, diced cucumber, chopped red onion, Kalamata olives, and crumbled feta cheese. This amalgamation of ingredients resembles a veritable mosaic of flavors intermingling harmoniously.

Incorporating Fresh Herbs:

To infuse the salad with a delightful Mediterranean freshness, I sprinkle in the finely chopped fresh parsley and mint. These aromatic herbs contribute an explosion of captivating aromas and delightful flavors, elevating the dish to new heights of culinary excellence.

Prepare the Dressing: Start by combining the freshly squeezed lemon juice and high-quality extra-virgin olive oil in a small bowl. This uncomplicated dressing adds a tangy and citrusy element that brings the whole dish together.

Mix and Season: Pour the delightful lemony dressing over the salad and gently mix all the ingredients until they are evenly coated. To enhance the flavor, add a pinch of salt and a sprinkle of freshly ground black pepper, adjusting the seasoning according to your preference.

Chill and Let it Settle: For optimal results, it is recommended to refrigerate the salad for approximately 30 minutes before serving. This allows the various flavors to blend harmoniously and the salad to cool down, creating a truly refreshing option, especially on a warm summer day.

Present and Indulge: When it is time to serve, artfully plate or elegantly place the Mediterranean Quinoa Salad into individual dishes or bowls. Whether enjoyed as a delightful lunch, a delectable side dish, or even a satisfying main course, this salad captures the essence of Mediterranean cuisine - bursting with freshness, vibrancy, and an array of enticing flavors. It is a culinary masterpiece that beautifully showcases a combination of ingredients, and sharing it with loved ones becomes an enchanting experience, knowing that each mouthful brings the essence of the Mediterranean sun.

Chapter 5: Satisfying Soups and Salads

Soup for the Soul

Authentic Greek Avgolemono

Preparing an authentic Greek Avgolemono soup is akin to embracing a timeless tradition that skillfully combines the vibrant flavors of lemon with the luxurious, velvety texture of eggs. Allow me to share my personal method for crafting this beloved Greek dish. To start, let's gather our ingredients:

- 4 cups of chicken or vegetable broth
- 1/2 cup of Arborio rice (or any other short-grain rice)

- *2 eggs*
- *Juice of 2-3 lemons (adjust according to your desired level of tartness)*
- *Salt and freshly ground black pepper to taste*
- *Fresh dill for optional garnish*

Now, let's embark on the journey of making this culinary masterpiece:

1. Preparing the Broth:
   In a pot, I gently bring the chicken or vegetable broth to a simmer over medium heat. It's crucial not to let it reach a rolling boil; a serene simmer is our objective.

2. Adding the Rice:
   Once our broth is simmering beautifully, I gracefully stir in the Arborio rice. This variety of rice works wonders for Avgolemono as its starch content imparts a delightful creaminess to the dish. I let it gently cook within the simmering broth until it reaches a tender state, which typically takes around 15-20 minutes.

3. Whisking the Eggs:
   In a separate bowl, I meticulously whisk the eggs until they become frothy and exhibit a light texture. It is vital to whisk them thoroughly to ensure easy integration into the soup, resulting in a harmonious consistency.

4. Incorporating the Lemon Juice:
   To the whisked eggs, I gradually add the juice of 2-3 lemons, taking into account my desired level of tartness. The lemon acts

as the very essence of Avgolemono, so I approach its quantity with careful consideration and precision.

5. Prepare the Eggs: This crucial step involves taking necessary precautions to prevent the eggs from curdling when added to the hot broth. To do this, I gently warm the eggs by slowly incorporating a ladleful of hot broth into the mixture of eggs and lemon. Throughout this process, I maintain a continuous whisking motion.

6. Incorporate the Egg-Lemon Mixture: Once the eggs have been properly tempered, I proceed by gradually pouring the mixture back into the simmering soup. I take care to stir the soup constantly, ensuring that the eggs and lemon juice blend seamlessly with the hot broth. This combination results in a delightful, velvety texture.

7. Simmer and Season: To allow the flavors to fully come together, I let the soup simmer for a few additional minutes. During this time, I take the opportunity to season the soup to taste by adding a pinch of salt and a dash of freshly ground black pepper.

8. Garnish and Serve: After the Avgolemono soup has reached its desired consistency, I ladle it into serving bowls. It can be enjoyed on its own, or for an added layer of flavor and freshness, it can be garnished with some freshly chopped dill.

Avgolemono is a timeless Greek classic that skillfully balances the zesty brightness of lemon with the comforting creaminess of the soup. Personally, I find joy in preparing and sharing this heartwarming dish, particularly on cold winter days or whenever I crave a taste of Greek tradition.

Tuscan White Bean and Kale Soup

Crafting Tuscan White Bean and Kale Soup is akin to creating a masterpiece of flavors, much like painting a picturesque Tuscan landscape. This unique approach to preparing the soup incorporates various ingredients that symbolize the rolling hills, vibrant greenery, and warm essence of Italy. Allow me to guide you through the process of making this comforting dish:

Ingredients:
- 2 tablespoons of high-quality olive oil
- Finely chopped onion
- Diced carrots
- Diced celery stalks
- Minced cloves of garlic
- A teaspoon of dried Italian herbs, including rosemary, thyme, and oregano
- Two cans (15 oz each) of cannellini beans, drained and rinsed
- Six cups of vegetable or chicken broth
- A bunch of kale, with stems removed and leaves chopped
- One bay leaf
- Salt and freshly ground black pepper, to taste
- Optional: Grated Parmesan cheese for garnish

Instructions:

1. Begin by sautéing the aromatics. Heat the olive oil in a large pot over medium heat. Add the finely chopped onion, diced carrots, and diced celery, and gently sauté them until they reach a tender and fragrant state. This essential step creates a flavor foundation for the soup.

2. Infuse the soup with aromatics. Stir in the minced garlic and the delightful blend of dried Italian herbs. This infusion adds a captivating aroma that will transport your senses to the heart of Tuscany.

3. Introduce the white beans to the pot. Add the drained and rinsed cannellini beans, which are a quintessential ingredient in Tuscan cuisine. These creamy white beans contribute a hearty and comforting element to the soup.

4. Add the Broth: Firstly, I pour the vegetable or chicken broth into the pot. The broth gracefully encompasses the beans and vegetables, forming the foundation of the soup with its delectable and savory taste.

5. Introduce the Kale: Next, I incorporate the finely chopped kale leaves into the mixture. Kale holds a special place in Tuscan cuisine, lending not only vibrant colors but also a wealth of nutritional value to the soup.

6. Bay Leaf and Seasoning: To enhance the flavor profile, I delicately place a bay leaf into the pot. A touch of salt and freshly ground black pepper is added to the soup, ensuring a perfect balance of flavors. These final additions create a rich and harmonious medley in the soup.

6. Simmer and Infuse: The soup is left to simmer gently over medium-low heat for approximately 20-30 minutes. This allows all the flavors to meld together and the kale to become tender. It resembles the unveiling of a mesmerizing Tuscan masterpiece.

7. Remove the Bay Leaf: Just before serving, I take care to remove the bay leaf. Its essence has been fully extracted, and it is time to bid farewell.

8. Serve and Garnish: When the moment arrives to relish the Tuscan White Bean and Kale Soup, I ladle it into bowls. For an extra touch of Italian authenticity, a sprinkle of grated Parmesan cheese on top can be added. This soup surpasses mere sustenance; it carries you on a journey to the sun-kissed Tuscan countryside with each spoonful. It possesses a comforting warmth, nourishment and wholesomeness that encapsulate the very essence of Italian culinary comfort. Buon !

Wholesome Salads

Classic Greek Salad

Creating a timeless Greek Salad is akin to assembling a vibrant tapestry of Mediterranean flavors, where each element serves as a lively piece in a grand masterpiece. Presenting a distinctive method to prepare this iconic dish:

Ingredients:

- *4 ripe tomatoes, sliced into wedges*
- *1 cucumber, thinly sliced*
- *1 red onion, finely sliced*
- *1 green bell pepper, cut into rings*
- *1/2 cup of pitted Kalamata olives*
- *200g of crumbled feta cheese*
- *1/4 cup of fresh oregano leaves*
- *Salt and freshly ground black pepper*

For the Dressing:
- *1/4 cup of extra-virgin olive oil*
- *2 tablespoons of red wine vinegar*
- *1 minced clove of garlic*
- *1 teaspoon of Dijon mustard*
- *1 teaspoon of honey (to add a touch of sweetness)*
- *Zest and juice of 1 lemon.*

Instructions:

Embrace the Mediterranean Palette: Start by arranging the tomato wedges in a circular arrangement on a spacious serving platter. This initial step is akin to setting the stage for a truly remarkable Mediterranean creation.

Cucumber Spirals: Craft delightful cucumber spirals using a vegetable peeler. These delicate ribbons add a playful and distinctive touch to your salad. Place them gracefully on top of the tomato wedges.

Onion Elegance: Scatter the thinly sliced red onion slices over the tomato and cucumber ensemble. The vibrant purple hue of the onions brings forth an artistic element to elevate the presentation.

Pepper Rings of Flavor: Integrate the green bell pepper rings amongst the other ingredients. They not only contribute vibrant colors but also offer a crisp and fresh sensation.

Kalamata Olives: Treat the placement of Kalamata olives with utmost care, as if they were precious gemstones, ensuring they appear throughout the salad. Their deep and rich flavor stands out as a true highlight.

Feta Crumbled Art: Crumble the feta cheese on top of the salad. This creamy and savory addition acts as an artist's brushstroke, enhancing the richness and texture.

Oregano Sprinkle: Sprinkle fresh oregano leaves over the salad, imparting a captivating and earthy aroma that distinctly commemorates Greek flavors.

Whisk the Dressing: In a small bowl, skillfully whisk together the exceptional combination of extra-virgin olive oil, red wine vinegar, minced garlic, Dijon mustard, honey, and the zest and juice of a lemon. This step can be compared to blending the colors on your artist's palette, resulting in a perfectly harmonized dressing.

Drizzle the Canvas: Generously drizzle the impeccably blended dressing all over the salad. This final touch acts as a unifying force that brings the flavors together, similar to applying varnish on a masterpiece.

Season with Love: Tenderly season your Greek Salad with a pinch of salt and a dash of freshly ground black pepper. The act of seasoning represents the signature of the artist.

Serve and Savor: Present your Classic Greek Salad as if showcasing an exhibit in a gallery, inviting your guests to truly relish the captivating flavors of the Mediterranean masterpiece you have created.

This Classic Greek Salad is not merely a dish; it is a meticulously crafted work of art, an ode to the delightful Mediterranean flavors, and a feast for all the senses. It offers a distinctive take on a timeless favorite that is bound to leave your guests marveling at your culinary prowess. Enjoy!

Mediterranean Couscous Salad

Crafting a Mediterranean Couscous Salad is akin to orchestrating a culinary masterpiece that unites a medley of textures, hues, and flavors. Allow me to present a unique approach for preparing this vibrant dish:

Ingredients:
- *1 cup of couscous*
- *1 1/4 cups of vegetable or chicken broth*
- *1 diced cucumber*
- *1 cup of halved cherry tomatoes*

- *1/2 finely chopped red onion*
- *1/2 cup of pitted and sliced Kalamata olives*
- *1/2 cup of crumbled feta cheese*
- *1/4 cup of chopped fresh mint leaves*
- *1/4 cup of chopped fresh parsley*

For the Dressing:
- *1/4 cup of extra-virgin olive oil*
- *2 tablespoons of red wine vinegar*
- *1 minced clove of garlic*
- *1 teaspoon of dried oregano*
- *Salt and freshly ground black pepper, to taste*
- *Zest and juice of 1 lemon*

Instructions:

Canvas of Fluffy Couscous: In a saucepan, I bring the vegetable or chicken broth to a boil. Then, I add the couscous, remove it from the heat, cover, and allow it to rest for approximately 5 minutes. After gently fluffing it with a fork, I am left with a blank canvas of light and airy couscous.

Tomato Gems: To infuse vibrant colors into my canvas, I scatter the cherry tomatoes, delicately halved like little jewels, throughout the couscous.

Crunchy Cucumber: I incorporate diced cucumber into the dish, reminiscent of crisp brushstrokes, adding a refreshing contrast to the couscous.

Elegant Onion: I carefully layer finely chopped red onion throughout the salad, akin to a delicate lace, contributing a subtle hint of sharpness.

Artistic Olives: Placing Kalamata olives, known for their deep, rich flavor, as bold and dark accents on the canvas, adds an artistic touch to the salad.

Poetic Feta Crumbles: Crumbling feta cheese over the salad is akin to adding poetic fragments that promise creamy, salty bursts of flavor.

Whispers of Mint and Parsley: I scatter fresh mint leaves and chopped parsley onto the salad like delicate whispers of freshness, imparting an aromatic and earthy essence to the dish.

Creating the Dressing: In a small bowl, I skillfully whisk together extra-virgin olive oil, red wine vinegar, minced garlic, dried oregano, salt, pepper, and the zest and juice of a lemon. This dressing acts as the conductor that harmonizes the flavors of the salad.

Precise Dressing Application: With precision, I drizzle the dressing over the couscous salad, ensuring that it coats each individual ingredient. It serves as the final brushstroke on this culinary masterpiece.

Gentle Tossing: With a gentle toss, I effortlessly blend and harmonize all the elements within the salad, creating a symphony of flavors, much like notes in a musical composition.

Presentation and Enjoyment: I proudly present this Mediterranean Couscous Salad as if it were a piece of art, a composition boasting a harmonious blend of colors, textures, and flavors waiting to be savored and admired.

This salad is not merely a dish; it is a culinary masterpiece that pays homage to the vibrant ingredients of the Mediterranean. It offers a unique twist on a classic, transforming a simple salad into a symphony that delights all the senses. Savor each and every bite!

Chapter 6: Savory Main Dishes

Seafood Sensations

Lemon-Garlic Grilled Shrimp

Preparing Lemon-Garlic Grilled Shrimp is akin to embarking on a voyage through the coastal realm, where the gentle whispers of the ocean meld harmoniously with the tantalizing fragrances of smoky grills. Allow me to elucidate my preferred method of crafting these delectable shrimp:

Essential Ingredients:
- *1 pound of exquisite, meticulously deveined large shrimp*
- *Minced essence of 3 cloves of garlic*
- *Aromatic zest and invigorating juice extracted from 2*

lemons
   - 2 tablespoons of the finest extra-virgin olive oil
   - 1 teaspoon of dried oregano, imbuing the dish with delightful herbal notes
   - An appropriate amount of salt and freshly ground black pepper, customized to match your discerning palate
   - Wooden skewers, abundantly soaked in rejuvenating water, to reliably coax grilling mastery
   With these resplendent ingredients at hand, let us embark upon our culinary odyssey.

Instructions:

Preparing the Shrimp: First, I ensure that the shrimp are peeled and deveined, leaving the tails intact for easy handling. In case I am using wooden skewers, I soak them in water to prevent them from burning when placed on the grill. Creating the Marinade: To make the marinade, I whisk together minced garlic, lemon zest, lemon juice, extra-virgin olive oil, dried oregano, salt, and freshly ground black pepper in a bowl. This marinade brings a burst of refreshing seaside flavor to the shrimp.

Marinating the Shrimp: I place the shrimp in either a resealable plastic bag or a shallow dish, and then carefully pour the marinade over them. I ensure that each shrimp is thoroughly coated in this zesty blend, offering an enticing invitation for them to soak up the Mediterranean flavors.

Resting and Infusing: The shrimp are left to marinate in the refrigerator for approximately 15-30 minutes. This brief resting period allows them to absorb the essence of lemon and garlic, enhancing their taste.

Preparing the Grill: While the shrimp are marinating, I preheat the grill to medium-high heat, aiming for the ideal grilling temperature.

Skewering the Shrimp: Next, I thread the marinated shrimp onto the wooden skewers, ensuring they are secure but not tightly packed. This not only makes grilling easier but also presents a visually appealing arrangement.

Grilling to Perfection: I place the shrimp skewers on the preheated grill, savoring the sound of their tantalizing sizzle and the aroma they release. I grill each side for approximately 2-3 minutes, or until the shrimp turn a beautiful pink color and become opaque. It's akin to witnessing the shrimp gracefully dance among the flames.

Serving with Joy: Once the Lemon-Garlic Grilled Shrimp has been cooked to perfection, with the grill's heat imparting a delicious kiss, I carefully remove them from the skewers and serve them with a smile. With every bite, I am transported to a Mediterranean seaside paradise.

These Lemon-Garlic Grilled Shrimp are more than just a dish; they embody the essence of summer, burst with refreshing coastal flavors, and serve as a reminder of how simple ingredients can create culinary wonders. Enjoy the delightful Mediterranean vibes with each succulent mouthful!

Mediterranean Baked Salmon

Preparing Mediterranean Baked Salmon is like taking a gastronomic voyage along the picturesque Mediterranean Sea. Let me guide you through the delectable creation of this exquisite dish using my personal recipe. Ingredients for this delightful culinary experience include:

- *4 succulent salmon filets*
  - *1 lemon, thinly sliced*
  - *1/4 cup of halved cherry tomatoes*
  - *1/4 cup of pitted Kalamata olives*
  - *2 cloves of garlic, finely minced*
  - *2 tablespoons of extra-virgin olive oil*
  - *1 teaspoon of dried oregano*
  - *Salt and freshly ground black pepper, to add finesse*
  - *Freshly chopped parsley, to garnish the dish perfectly*
  Now, let's embark on the journey of creating the Mediterranean Baked Salmon!

Instructions:
  Begin by preheating the oven to 375°F (190°C). As the oven warms up, the delightful aroma of Mediterranean flavors fills the air, creating an atmosphere of anticipation. Now, let's prepare the salmon for our culinary masterpiece.

Take the salmon filets and place them carefully on a baking sheet that's been lined with parchment paper. This step is akin to preparing a canvas for a work of art. To enhance the richness of the salmon, drizzle some extra-virgin olive oil over the filets. Then, season them with minced garlic, dried oregano, salt, and freshly ground black pepper. These well-balanced seasonings bring out the natural flavors of the salmon, adding depth and complexity.

Now, it's time to add layers of refreshing elements to our dish. Place thin slices of lemon over the salmon, allowing their tangy, citrusy essence to infuse into the fish. Next, scatter halved cherry tomatoes, resembling little drops of Mediterranean sunshine, over the salmon.

To amplify the taste profile even more, generously scatter pitted Kalamata olives around the salmon. These olives, with their briny flavor, provide a contrasting depth that complements the other ingredients perfectly.

To seal in all the flavors and textures, gently fold up the sides of the parchment paper, creating a secure "packet." This technique ensures that the salmon and the accompanying Mediterranean ingredients are cocooned together, ready to transform into a symphony of flavors within the oven.

With care and attention, place the baking sheet into the pre-heated oven and let it bake for approximately 15-20 minutes. Keep a watchful eye until the salmon flakes easily when probed with a fork. This transformative process within the oven magically blends all the components, creating a harmonious culinary orchestra.

The time has come to unveil this delectable delight. Slowly and cautiously, unfold the parchment paper packet, unleashing the enticing aroma of the Mediterranean Baked Salmon. Before serving this masterpiece, give it a final touch of freshness and color by garnishing with freshly chopped parsley. This addition resembles the finishing stroke on a culinary canvas, enhancing both the visual appeal and the overall taste experience.

Now, it's time to savor the fruits of your labor. With a sense of accomplishment, serve the Mediterranean Baked Salmon and savor each bite. As you indulge, you are transported to the picturesque coastlines of the Mediterranean, where the refreshing sea breeze merges with the vibrant flavors.

This dish isn't merely a meal. It's an escape to the Mediterranean, a celebration of simplicity and freshness, and a reminder of the pleasures that can be crafted right in the comfort of your own kitchen.

Poultry Pleasures

Roasted Lemon and Herb Chicken

Crafting a scrumptious Roasted Lemon and Herb Chicken is akin to orchestrating a harmonious blend of flavors right in the comfort of your own kitchen. Allow me to share my personal approach to preparing this delectable dish. Ingredients:

- *1 complete chicken (weighing approximately 4-5 pounds)*
  - *1 lemon*
  - *3-4 cloves of garlic*
  - *Sprigs of fresh rosemary*
  - *Sprigs of fresh thyme*
  - *Salt and freshly ground black pepper*
  - *Olive oil*

Instructions:

Begin by preheating the oven to 375°F (190°C). As the oven warms up, the tantalizing scent of aromatic herbs and lemon fills the air, creating a sense of anticipation. Next, prepare the chicken by patting it dry with paper towels. This step is crucial as it helps the skin become beautifully crispy during the roasting process. It's like preparing a blank canvas for a masterpiece of flavors.

Now it's time to season the chicken generously. Sprinkle salt and freshly ground black pepper both inside and outside of the chicken. This step forms the foundation of flavor that will elevate the entire dish. To enhance the taste, stuff the chicken cavity with lemon halves, whole garlic cloves, fresh rosemary sprigs, and fresh thyme sprigs. This combination of herbs and citrus creates a symphony of flavors that will permeate the chicken.

For an aesthetically pleasing and evenly cooked chicken, securely tie the chicken's legs together using kitchen twine. This adds a touch of elegance and ensures a perfectly roasted shape.

Drizzle a small amount of olive oil over the chicken's skin and massage it gently with your hands. This creates a glossy finish and helps the skin turn wonderfully crisp and golden during the roasting process.

Now it's time to place the chicken on a roasting rack in a baking pan. This step is like centering the star of the show on a stage. The chicken is ready to be roasted in the preheated oven for approximately 1.5 to 2 hours, or until the internal temperature reaches 165°F (74°C) and the skin achieves a beautiful golden brown color.

To maintain moisture and flavor, occasionally baste the chicken with the pan juices while it roasts in the oven. This ensures that every bite remains succulent and full of taste.

Once the roasting is complete, allow the chicken to rest for about 15 minutes. This allows the flavorful juices to redistribute throughout the meat, resulting in a juicy and succulent texture.

Now it's time to carve the Roasted Lemon and Herb Chicken. Serve each slice with the pan juices infused with lemon and herbs. Every mouthful bursts with a symphony of flavors, as the herbs and citrus create a delightful harmony. This dish is more than just a meal; it's a culinary masterpiece, demonstrating the magic that unfolds when simple yet high-quality ingredients come together. It's a joy to prepare and a pleasure to indulge in.

Moroccan-Inspired Turkey Tagine

Embark on a tantalizing journey to the heart of North Africa with the creation of a delightful Moroccan-Inspired Turkey Tagine. Here's an exceptional and innovative method to prepare this comforting and aromatic dish:

Ingredients:
- 1.5 pounds of succulent turkey breast or thigh, skillfully cut into delectable chunks
- 2 tablespoons of premium quality olive oil
- Finely diced onion, adding a burst of flavor
- Minced garlic, enhancing the aromatic essence
- 2 teaspoons of ground cumin, enriching the dish with its distinctive taste
- 1 teaspoon of ground coriander, lending its subtle notes
- 1 teaspoon of ground cinnamon, infusing a delightful warmth
- A teaspoon of paprika, adding a mild kick
- Half a teaspoon of ground ginger, intensifying the culinary experience
- A quarter teaspoon of cayenne pepper (adjust according to your preferred level of heat)
- One can of drained and rinsed chickpeas (14 oz), perfectly harmonizing with the other ingredients
- A can of diced tomatoes (14 oz), contributing to the exquisite blend
- One cup of chicken or vegetable broth, further enhancing the taste

- Half a cup of chopped, dried apricots which provide a hint of sweetness

- A quarter cup of thinly sliced almonds, contributing a delightful crunch

- A dash of salt and freshly ground black pepper, to tastefully season

- For the finishing touch, fresh cilantro to elegantly garnish the dish

Instructions:

To begin, I preheat either my tagine or a large, heavy-bottomed pot over medium-high heat. The kitchen is instantly filled with the tantalizing aroma of Moroccan spices. Next, I add a drizzle of olive oil to the heated tagine and proceed to brown the pieces of turkey on all sides. This crucial step helps to lock in the juices and infuse the meat with a delicious depth of flavor. Once the turkey is perfectly browned, I carefully set it aside.

Using the same tagine, I sauté finely chopped onions and minced garlic until they soften and release a delightful fragrance, reminiscent of the opening notes of a spice-filled symphony. At this point, I incorporate ground cumin, ground coriander, ground cinnamon, paprika, ground ginger, and a hint of cayenne pepper into the sautéed onions and garlic. As these aromatic spices mingle, their enchanting scents fill the air, capturing my senses.

Now it's time to reintroduce the seared turkey back into the tagine, ensuring that every piece is thoroughly coated in the fragrant spice blend. To create a luscious base, I pour in diced tomatoes and either chicken or vegetable broth, akin to the canvas that provides the backdrop for a beautiful Moroccan mosaic. To enhance both texture and a sweet-tangy balance, I add chickpeas and chopped dried apricots, which glisten like gems amidst the savory goodness of the dish.

Allowing everything to simmer and meld together over low heat for approximately 30-40 minutes, I occasionally stir to ensure that each ingredient harmonizes perfectly. In a separate pan, I toast slivered almonds until they turn a golden hue and exude a fragrant aroma, acting as the final embellishment, much like the vibrant strokes of color on a masterpiece.

As a finishing touch, I garnish the magnificent Moroccan-Inspired Turkey Tagine with the toasted almonds and sprigs of fresh cilantro. Each serving resembles a beautifully composed work of Moroccan art. This dish goes beyond being a mere meal; it transports you on a sensory expedition to the bustling souks and fragrant spice markets of Morocco. With every delectable bite, the combination of savory, sweet, and spicy flavors whisks you away to the enchanting landscape of North Africa. Immerse yourself in the magic of Moroccan cuisine and enjoy this extraordinary culinary experience!

Chapter 7: Hearty Vegetarian Fare

Veggie-Centric Creations

Eggplant Parmesan

Preparing Eggplant Parmesan involves crafting a delectable Italian dish that offers a blissful combination of flavors and textures. Here's a step-by-step guide on how to create this enticing delight:

Ingredients:
  - *2 substantial eggplants*
  - *2 cups of versatile all-purpose flour*
  - *3 large eggs*
  - *2 cups of breadcrumbs (preferably Italian-style)*
  - *2 cups of marinara sauce*

- 2 cups of shredded mozzarella cheese
- 1/2 cup of grated Parmesan cheese
- 1/4 cup of freshly chopped basil leaves
- Salt and freshly ground black pepper, to enhance the taste
- Olive oil for frying
- Fresh basil leaves for garnish (optional)

How to Prepare Eggplants:

Begin by slicing the eggplants into 1/4-inch thick rounds. Sprinkle a little salt on both sides of the slices and allow them to sit in a colander for approximately 30 minutes. This will help remove any excess moisture and bitterness. Afterward, gently pat them dry using paper towels.

Setting up a Breading Station: Set up a breading station by using three separate shallow dishes. Place the flour in one dish, beaten eggs in another, and breadcrumbs in the third dish. This will make it easier to coat the eggplant slices.

Breading the Eggplant: Take each slice of eggplant and coat it first in flour, then dip it into the beaten eggs, and finally coat it in breadcrumbs, pressing lightly to ensure they adhere. Place the breaded slices on a baking sheet.

Frying the Eggplant: In a large skillet, heat approximately 1/4 inch of olive oil over medium-high heat. Once the oil is hot, add the breaded eggplant slices in batches and fry until they turn golden brown on both sides, which should take about 2-3 minutes per side. Place the fried slices on paper towels to drain off any excess oil.

Preheating the Oven: Preheat your oven to 375°F (190°C).

Assembling the Layers: In a baking dish, spread a thin layer of marinara sauce. Place a single layer of fried eggplant slices on top of the sauce. Sprinkle it with mozzarella and Parmesan cheese, and add a few chopped fresh basil leaves. Continue layering with sauce, eggplant, cheese, and basil until all the ingredients are used, finishing with a layer of cheese on top.

Baking and Melting: Cover the baking dish with aluminum foil and bake in the preheated oven for approximately 20-25 minutes. This will allow the cheese to melt and the flavors to meld together.

Optional Crispy Top: If you desire a golden and crispy top, you can remove the foil and broil the dish for an additional 2-3 minutes, but be sure to keep a close eye on it to prevent burning.

Serving and Garnishing: Allow the Eggplant Parmesan to rest for a few minutes before serving. You can garnish it with fresh basil leaves if desired.

This Eggplant Parmesan is more than just a meal; it is a comforting Italian classic with layers of crispy eggplant, flavorful tomato sauce, and delectable melted cheese. Every bite is a savory delight that is perfect for a family dinner or to impress your guests. Enjoy!

Spanakopita (Spinach Pie)

Creating Spanakopita, the beloved and renowned Greek spinach pie, involves a culinary process that artfully combines layers of delicate, flaky pastry with a delectable filling of savory spinach. Here, we present a distinctive way to meticulously craft this mouthwatering dish:

Ingredients:

For the Filling:
- 2 pounds of fresh spinach, thoroughly washed and finely chopped
- 1 cup of crumbled feta cheese
- 1 cup of ricotta cheese
- 1/2 cup of grated Parmesan cheese
- 1 small onion, finely diced
- 3 cloves of garlic, minced
- A handful of freshly chopped dill
- Olive oil for sautéing
- Salt and freshly ground black pepper, to enhance the flavors
- A dash of ground nutmeg for a subtle hint of warmth

For the Layers:
- 1 package of phyllo dough (typically containing 18 sheets)
- 1 cup of melted butter or olive oil, for brushing the layers

Instructions:

Preparing the Spinach: To start, sauté the finely chopped spinach in a pan with a drizzle of olive oil until it becomes wilted and releases its moisture. Next, remove any excess liquid, squeeze out the remaining moisture from the spinach, and finely chop it.

Sautéing the Aromatics: In the same pan, sauté the finely chopped onion and minced garlic until they become fragrant and turn golden. This aromatic base adds depth to the filling.

Creating the Filling: In a large mixing bowl, combine the sautéed spinach, crumbled feta cheese, ricotta cheese, grated Parmesan cheese, chopped fresh dill, sautéed onion, and garlic. Season this mixture with salt, freshly ground black pepper, and a pinch of ground nutmeg. The combination of these ingredients is akin to composing a symphony of flavors.

Preparing the Phyllo Dough: Unroll the phyllo dough and cover it with a clean kitchen towel to prevent it from drying out while you work. The phyllo dough serves as the canvas for our savory masterpiece.

Layering and Brushing: Take one sheet of phyllo dough and place it on a baking sheet, then brush it with melted butter or olive oil. Repeat this process, layering and brushing each sheet, to create a flaky and golden crust.

Adding the Filling: Spread a generous portion of the spinach and cheese mixture onto the layered phyllo dough. This is like adding a savory mosaic to the canvas.

Folding and Layering: Fold the edges of the phyllo dough over the filling to create a neat package. Then, layer more sheets of phyllo on top, brushing each one with butter or olive oil. Repeat this process until all the filling is used.

Baking to Perfection: Preheat the oven to 350°F (175°C) and bake the Spanakopita for approximately 45-50 minutes, or until it turns beautifully golden brown and the filling is set.

Cooling and Slicing: Allow the Spanakopita to cool for a bit before slicing it into squares or triangles. This step helps the layers to set and results in a flaky and savory masterpiece.

Serving with a Smile: Serve this unique Spanakopita with a smile, knowing that each bite is a delightful combination of flaky pastry and a savory spinach and cheese filling. It's not just a dish; it's a delightful blend of textures and flavors that captures the essence of Greek cuisine. Perfect as either an appetizer or a main course, this dish is a testament to the artistry of Mediterranean cooking. Enjoy!

Plant-Based Protein Powder

Chickpea and Spinach Stew

Crafting a Chickpea and Spinach Stew is akin to conducting an exquisite symphony of flavors, where each element harmoniously contributes to the overall composition. Allow me to present a distinctive approach to preparing this nourishing and satisfying dish:

Ingredients:
- 2 cans (15 oz each) of chickpeas, thoroughly drained and rinsed
- 1 finely chopped large onion
- 3 minced cloves of garlic
- 1 diced red bell pepper
- 1 teaspoon of ground cumin
- 1 teaspoon of ground coriander
- 1/2 teaspoon of smoked paprika
- 1/4 teaspoon of cayenne pepper (adjust according to desired level of spiciness)
- 1 can (14 oz) of diced tomatoes
- 4 cups of fresh spinach, finely chopped
- 4 cups of vegetable broth
- 2 tablespoons of olive oil
- Salt and freshly ground black pepper, to taste
- Fresh lemon wedges, for garnish
- Fresh cilantro leaves, for garnish
Now, let's embark on the culinary journey of transforming these ingredients into a divine Chickpea and Spinach Stew.

Instructions:

Begin by heating olive oil in a large pot over medium heat. Next, add the finely chopped onion, minced garlic, and diced red bell pepper to the pot. Sauté them until they become tender and fragrant, creating a delicious base for the stew.

After that, add ground cumin, ground coriander, smoked paprika, and a touch of cayenne pepper to the sautéed ingredients. Stirring in these spices is akin to adding musical notes to enhance the symphony of flavors in the stew. Now it's time to introduce the drained and rinsed chickpeas and the can of diced tomatoes to the pot. These components contribute a robust texture and a tangy sweetness to the dish.

Pour in the vegetable broth, which envelops the chickpeas and tomatoes like a comforting melody. The broth serves as the heart and soul of the stew. Allow the stew to simmer for about 15-20 minutes to allow the flavors to meld together harmoniously. During this time, use an immersion blender to partially puree the stew. This step creates a velvety texture while still retaining some whole chickpeas for added depth. Gently fold in the chopped fresh spinach, letting it wilt gracefully into the stew. The vibrant green of the spinach adds a pop of color and a healthy dose of nutrients.

Season the Chickpea and Spinach Stew with salt and freshly ground black pepper, adjusting the seasonings to your liking. The act of seasoning is similar to fine-tuning the notes of a melody, enhancing the overall taste experience. Serve the stew hot, garnished with fresh lemon wedges and cilantro leaves.

The addition of lemon provides a zesty burst of flavor, while the cilantro acts as the perfect finishing touch on this culinary masterpiece.

This stew is more than just a dish; it is a delightful fusion of spices and textures, a symphony of flavors that is both satisfying and nourishing. It is ideal for a comforting meal on a chilly evening and showcases the beauty of vegetarian cuisine. Indulge in the symphony of taste!

Falafel with Tzatziki Sauce

Creating Falafel with Tzatziki Sauce is akin to composing a harmonious culinary symphony, where contrasting textures and flavors combine to create a delightful experience. Here's an innovative technique to craft this timeless delicacy from the Mediterranean region:

Ingredients:

For the Falafel:
- *2 cups of dried chickpeas*
- *1 small onion, roughly chopped*
- *4 cloves of garlic, finely minced*
- *1/4 cup of freshly chopped parsley*
- *1/4 cup of freshly chopped cilantro*
- *1 teaspoon of ground cumin*
- *1 teaspoon of ground coriander*

- *1/4 teaspoon of cayenne pepper*
- *1 teaspoon of baking powder*
- *Salt and freshly ground black pepper, to taste*
- *Vegetable oil for frying*

For the Tzatziki Sauce:
- *1 cup of Greek yogurt*
- *1/2 cucumber, grated and squeezed to remove excess moisture*
- *2 cloves of garlic, finely minced*
- *2 tablespoons of freshly chopped dill*
- *2 tablespoons of freshly chopped mint*
- *Juice of 1 lemon*
- *Salt and freshly ground black pepper, to taste*

By delicately blending these ingredients, we embark on a culinary adventure that results in a mouthwatering dish. Let's dive into the process:

Instructions: To Make the Falafel:

1. Prepare the Chickpeas: Start by soaking the dried chickpeas in water overnight. This process hydrates them and prepares them for blending

2. Blend the Ingredients: In a food processor, combine the soaked chickpeas, roughly chopped onion, minced garlic, fresh parsley, fresh cilantro, ground cumin, ground coriander, cayenne pepper, baking powder, salt, and freshly ground black pepper. Blend until the mixture is coarse but well combined, akin to a finely orchestrated musical composition

3. Form the Falafel Patties: Shape the mixture into small patties or balls, like crafting little falafel masterpieces

4. Fry to Perfection: Heat vegetable oil to 350°F (175°C) in a deep skillet. Carefully place the falafel into the hot oil and fry until they turn golden brown and achieve a satisfying crispy texture, resembling a skillfully played crescendo

5. Drain and Cool: Once cooked, remove the falafel and place them on paper towels to drain any excess oil. Allow them to cool, much like giving music notes a moment of rest.

To Make the Tzatziki Sauce:

1. Prepare the Base: In a mixing bowl, combine Greek yogurt, grated cucumber that has been squeezed dry, minced garlic, fresh dill, fresh mint, and the juice of a lemon. This step creates a refreshing and harmonious foundation note

2. Season with Precision: Add salt and freshly ground black pepper to the Tzatziki sauce, adjusting the seasoning according to your taste. Adjusting the seasoning is comparable to finely tuning the melody of the sauce

3. Serve in Harmony: Serve the crispy, golden falafel alongside the cool and creamy Tzatziki sauce. Each bite will be a duet of textures and flavors, where the savory richness of the falafel is perfectly balanced by the refreshing and tangy notes of the sauce. This combination creates a culinary composition, a fusion of textures and flavors that is both satisfying and invigorating. It embodies the harmonious essence of Mediterranean cuisine and is guaranteed to delight your taste buds. Enjoy the symphony of flavors!

Chapter 8: Sides and Accompaniments

~~~

Mediterranean Rice Pilaf

I am delighted to share my recipe for Mediterranean Rice Pilaf, a delectable and aromatic rice dish that harmoniously combines long-grain rice with a medley of fragrant herbs, spices, and occasionally toasted nuts. This versatile side dish complements an array of Mediterranean-inspired main courses flawlessly. Now, let me guide you through my personal approach to preparing this delightful Mediterranean Rice Pilaf.

Ingredients:
  - 1 cup of long-grain white rice
  - 2 cups of chicken or vegetable broth
~~~

- *2 tablespoons of olive oil*
- *Finely chopped small onion*
- *Minced cloves of garlic*
- *1/2 cup of assorted Mediterranean herbs (such as freshly chopped parsley, dill, and mint)*
- *Optional: 1/4 cup of toasted pine nuts or slivered almonds*
- *1 teaspoon of ground cumin*
- *1/2 teaspoon of ground coriander*
- *Salt and freshly ground black pepper, to taste*
- *Fresh lemon wedges, for serving*
Let's begin the culinary journey!

Instructions:

Begin by rinsing the rice with cold water until the water runs clear. This step helps remove excess starch, resulting in light and fluffy grains. Once rinsed, drain the rice and set it aside.

Next, heat olive oil in a large skillet over medium heat. Add finely chopped onions and minced garlic, sautéing them until they become soft and translucent.

This process resembles the beginning notes of a delightful melody. To infuse the dish with flavors, incorporate ground cumin and ground coriander into the sautéed aromatics.

Allow the spices to toast for a minute or two, releasing their warm and earthy fragrance.

Now, incorporate the rinsed and drained rice into the skillet, stirring often to toast it until it becomes slightly translucent. This toasting is akin to a gentle crescendo in the melody of the dish.

Pour in chicken or vegetable broth and include a mixture of Mediterranean herbs such as fresh parsley, dill, and mint. Each herb contributes a unique note to bring the dish alive.

Season the mixture with salt and freshly ground black pepper, adjusting to taste. Bring it to a boil, then reduce the heat and cover, allowing it to simmer for approximately 15-20 minutes. During this time, the rice absorbs the flavors, much like a melody reaching its peak.

Once the rice is cooked and the liquid is absorbed, fluff it with a fork. Optional toppings, such as toasted pine nuts or slivered almonds, add a delightful crunch to the finishing notes of the melody.

When serving the Mediterranean Rice Pilaf, accompany it with fresh lemon wedges. This permits each person to add a bright and zesty note to their portion by squeezing lemon juice over it.

This Mediterranean Rice Pilaf is not just a mere side dish; it is a culinary composition, a symphony of flavors that pairs perfectly with a wide range of Mediterranean-inspired meals. Its versatility and aromatic quality make it a wonderful addition to any table. Enjoy the harmonious flavors!

Roasted Vegetables with Balsamic Glaze

I love indulging in the exquisite delicacy that is Roasted Vegetables with Balsamic Glaze. This delightful dish beautifully marries the inherent sweetness of oven-roasted vegetables with a luscious and tangy balsamic reduction. The end result is a flawless amalgamation of flavors and textures that will tantalize your taste buds. If you're curious about the process, allow me to walk you through how I prepare this magnificent dish. To begin with, you will need an array of assorted vegetables. Opt for vibrant bell peppers, succulent zucchini, juicy cherry tomatoes, enticing red onions, and tender asparagus.

In order to accomplish the perfect combination of flavors, make sure to have some high-quality olive oil on hand, along with a pinch of salt and some freshly ground black pepper. These simple seasonings will undoubtedly elevate the taste profile of your roasted vegetables.

To achieve that distinctive tangy glaze, you'll want to acquire some top-notch balsamic vinegar. Additionally, you may choose to add a touch of sweetness using either honey or maple syrup. The infusion of these ingredients will add depth and complexity to your creation.

Finally, if you desire an extra touch of elegance, consider garnishing your dish with fresh herbs such as aromatic rosemary, fragrant thyme, or even some refreshing basil. This optional addition will not only enhance the visual appeal but also lend a subtle burst of fragrance to the overall experience.

Embrace the art of culinary exploration and give Roasted Vegetables with Balsamic Glaze a try. Treat yourself to a culinary masterpiece that combines the finest ingredients, harmonious flavors, and delectable textures.

Instructions:

Begin by preheating the oven to a temperature of 425°F (220°C). As the oven heats up, a delightful anticipation fills the kitchen, infusing it with a comforting warmth.

Next, it's time to prepare the vegetables, selecting a diverse assortment akin to an artist carefully choosing a vibrant palette of colors. Depending on their size and variety, I either cut them into bite-sized pieces or leave them whole.

Moving on, I take a generous amount of olive oil and drizzle it over the vegetables in a spacious mixing bowl. With my hands, I ensure that every piece is evenly coated, resembling a sacred act of anointing, infusing each morsel with exquisite flavor.

To enhance their natural essence, I season the vegetables with a liberal amount of salt and freshly ground black pepper. This allows their inherent flavors to emerge and captivate the senses, like a captivating melody demanding attention.

Once fully seasoned, I carefully arrange the vegetables in a single, uniform layer on a baking sheet, ensuring they have ample space for even roasting. With great care, I place the baking sheet into the preheated oven, embarking on a culinary journey where they will transform into tender, slightly caramelized treasures.

While the vegetables undergo their delectable metamorphosis, it is the perfect opportunity to prepare the balsamic glaze. In a small saucepan, I combine balsamic vinegar with a touch of honey or maple syrup, bringing the mixture to a gentle simmer. Slowly, the glaze reduces by half, thickening into a luscious symphony of sweet and tangy flavors.

As the vegetables are near completion, I eagerly await their arrival. Once they are done roasting, I drizzle the indulgent balsamic glaze over them, creating a cascading masterpiece of flavors, much like a crescendo in a captivating musical performance.

Gently, I toss the vegetables to ensure each one is coated with the luxurious glaze, allowing for a harmonious infusion of flavors. If I have the pleasure of having fresh herbs such as rosemary, thyme, or basil at hand, I sprinkle them delicately over the roasted vegetables, acting as the final delicate notes in a delightful melody, adding a touch of freshness and charm. With enthusiasm and a smile on my face,

I proudly present the Roasted Vegetables with Balsamic Glaze, knowing that each bite offers a delightful combination of savory roasted goodness and the elegant sweetness of the glaze.

This dish is not just a mere side, but rather a masterpiece of culinary composition, seamlessly harmonizing flavors and textures. The roasted vegetables embody a vibrant orchestra, while the balsamic glaze assumes the role of the conductor, coaxing out their harmonious notes with finesse. In conclusion, indulge in this exquisite medley of flavors, savoring each moment and allowing yourself to be enveloped by the symphony of tastes.

Quinoa Tabbouleh

Quinoa Tabbouleh presents a delightful variation of the traditional Middle Eastern salad, which is conventionally prepared with bulgur wheat. In this distinct rendition, bulgur is substituted with quinoa, providing a gluten-free and protein-rich option. Now, let's discover a unique approach to crafting Quinoa Tabbouleh.

Here are the essential ingredients:

1 cup of quinoa,
2 cups of water,
2 cups of finely chopped fresh parsley,
1 cup of finely chopped fresh mint leaves, 1 cup of quartered cherry tomatoes,
1 diced cucumber,
1/2 red onion finely chopped,
3 tablespoons of olive oil, juice extracted from
2 lemons, and salt and freshly ground black pepper to enhance the flavor according to personal preference.

Instructions:

Begin by rinsing the quinoa under cold water to cleanse it of any bitterness. Afterwards, combine the quinoa with 2 cups of water in a saucepan and bring it to a boil. Let it simmer for approximately 15 minutes or until the quinoa has absorbed the water and become tender. Once cooked, use a fork to fluff the quinoa and allow it to cool.

While the quinoa is cooking, finely chop the fresh parsley and mint leaves. These vibrant herbs bring freshness and a vivid pop of color to the dish. Next, prepare the vegetables by dicing the cucumber, quartering the cherry tomatoes, and finely chopping the red onion. These ingredients come together to create a harmonious mix of textures and flavors.

In a large bowl, combine the cooked and cooled quinoa with the chopped herbs, diced cucumber, quartered tomatoes, and finely chopped red onion. Think of this step as assembling a group of musical instruments, each with its own unique qualities, to create a harmonious ensemble.

As a conductor's baton unites different sections of an orchestra, drizzle olive oil and freshly squeezed lemon juice over the salad to bring all the ingredients together with a refreshing and zesty melody. Season the salad with salt and freshly ground black pepper, fine-tuning the flavors to perfection.

Gently toss the Quinoa Tabbouleh, ensuring that all the elements are well mixed and harmonized, just like blending different musical instruments into a beautiful composition.

Allow the salad to chill in the refrigerator for at least 30 minutes.

This time allows the flavors to meld together and reach their peak, creating a truly delightful melody.

Serve the Quinoa Tabbouleh with a joyful heart, knowing that each bite is a symphony of textures and tastes. This unique twist on a classic salad offers a wholesome and gluten-free melody of Mediterranean flavors. It is more than just a salad; it is a culinary composition, seamlessly blending textures and herbs to bring a modern twist to traditional Tabbouleh. Enjoy this delightful medley of flavors as a refreshing side dish or a light meal on its own.

Chapter 9: Sweet Mediterranean Endings

Decadent Desserts

Baklava

Baklava, a cherished dessert in Mediterranean cuisine, is a delectable pastry known for its decadence. This exquisite treat is crafted by delicately layering thin phyllo dough with a delightful mixture of chopped nuts, perfectly complemented by a luscious syrup or honey. The art of creating baklava is akin to conducting a symphony, blending sweetness and crispiness to create a masterpiece.

The Foundation of Baklava: At the core of baklava lies the essence of phyllo dough. In Greek, "phyllo" translates to "leaf," reflecting its nature as paper-thin pastry dough. Each layer is carefully brushed with melted butter, adding a crispy and golden touch once baked. As the layers are painstakingly stacked one by one, they give rise to a delicate and flaky texture.

Nutty Pleasures: Nestled between the layers of phyllo dough, a mixture of nuts is generously spread. Often including walnuts, pistachios, and almonds, these nuts are coarsely chopped to lend a delightful crunch. Completing the symphony of flavors, some variations of baklava incorporate a hint of spice. Time-honored choices such as cinnamon and cloves bless the nuts with their warm and aromatic essence.

Creating an Elegant Presentation: Following the layering of phyllo and nut mixture, the pastry is typically sliced into exquisite diamond-shaped or square pieces. This not only showcases the ultimate sophistication of baklava but also ensures that the syrup or honey can evenly permeate every nook and cranny, amplifying the taste sensation.

The Finishing Touch: Once prepared, the baklava is gently placed in the oven, where it undergoes its transformation. The phyllo layers gradually turn a majestic golden brown, achieving the desired crispiness. The butter plays its part in creating a flaky texture, while the nuts toast, infusing the delicacy with enhanced flavor and a satisfying crunch.

Delightful Delicacy: Once the baklava emerges from the heated oven, a steaming syrup concocted from sugar, water, and lemon juice is generously poured over it. The layers eagerly soak up the hot syrup, resulting in a saccharine and sticky glaze. To enhance its sweetness, a drizzle of honey can also be added on top.

Absorption and Resting: The baklava is given time to rest and absorb the syrup, transforming into a lavish, rich, and decadent delight. This period of cooling is crucial for the layers to settle and attain their distinctive texture.

Serving: Baklava can be served in petite, bite-sized portions, making it an ideal choice for communal enjoyment. It is often adorned with additional nuts, presenting an aesthetic vision as captivating as its taste.

Baklava stands out as a dessert of unparalleled uniqueness, with an interplay of textures and flavors. The crispy and buttery phyllo dough layers perfectly contrast with the sweetness of the syrupy interior. The inclusion of nuts provides a delightful crunch, while the spices contribute depth and complexity. It is a harmonious symphony of flavors that not only pleases the palate but also captivates the senses with its visually artistic presentation. Indulging in a piece of baklava mirrors the experience of savoring a luxurious and harmonious melody within the Mediterranean culinary tradition.

How to make Baklava

Baklava's layers of phyllo dough, spiced nuts, and honeyed syrup are like layers of a sweet and nutty masterpiece. Here's a creative way to make this delicious dessert:

Components:

Regarding Filling:
Two cups of finely chopped mixed nuts, including pistachios, almonds, and walnuts
1/2 cup of sugar, granulated
one tsp finely ground cinnamon
1/4 teaspoon of cloves, ground

About the Layers of Phyllo:

One packet of phyllo dough, which typically has eighteen sheets
One cup and two sticks of melted unsalted butter

Regarding Syrup:
1 cup of sugar, granulated
half a cup of water
halved cup honey
One stick of cinnamon
2–3 complete cloves
A couple of lemon zest strips

Guidelines:

Get the Filling Ready:

I begin by putting the finely chopped mixed nuts in a bowl with sugar, ground cloves, and ground cinnamon. This mixture, which adds notes of sweetness, nuttiness, and spice, is similar to the center of a baklava.

Warm up the oven:
The oven is preheated to 350°F, or 175°C. The Baklava is about to transform.

Get the Phyllo Dough Ready:
To prevent it from drying out, I unroll the phyllo dough and cover it with a damp kitchen towel. To get ready for layering, I quickly brush melted butter on a baking dish.

Butter and Layer:
I take one sheet of phyllo dough and brush it with more melted butter before placing it in the buttered baking dish. I continue layering and buttering until about half of the sheets are used. It's similar to painting the backdrop for our masterwork of Baklava.

Include the Nut Blend:
I doped the phyllo layers with a good helping of the nut mixture. It's like adding the flavor and texture of the artwork's core.

Proceed with Layering:
I cover the phyllo with additional layers, brushing each one with melted butter. I then carry out the same procedure with the remaining nuts, resulting in layers of artistic crispness and nutty flavor.

Complete the Layers:

Using the remaining phyllo sheets, I complete the Baklava by brushing the top sheet with additional butter. It's similar to finishing touches on a masterpiece.

Cut Diamond-Shape:
I gently cut the Baklava into square or diamond shapes with a sharp knife so that the layers could equally absorb the syrup. The cuts resemble precisely timed notes in music.

Bake until done:
Baklava is placed in the preheated oven and baked for 45 to 50 minutes, or until it is crisp and golden brown, resembling the final crescendo of a lovely melody.

Get the syrup ready.
I make the syrup as the Baklava bakes. I mix sugar, water, honey, a cinnamon stick, whole cloves, and lemon zest in a saucepan. I simmered it for ten minutes or so, turning it into a spiced and sweet syrup.

Dip in Syrup:
I immediately covered the Baklava with the hot syrup after taking it out of the oven. Every bite is infused with warmth and sweetness as the syrup seeps into the layers.

Set and Cool:
I let the Baklava cool all the way down so that, like a piece of music, the flavors would combine and the layers would solidify.

Present with a Garnish:
Knowing that every bite of the Baklava is a symphony of

crispy layers, sweet syrup, and spiced nuts, I present it with gusto. It's a decadent and unusual dessert that will tickle your taste buds.

Baklava embodies the essence of Mediterranean sweets and is more than just a dessert. It's a culinary composition, a symphony of layers and flavors. Savor this delightful work of art!

Orange and Almond Cake

Creating an Orange and Almond Cake is similar to producing a nutty, sunny, and citrus-flavored cake that is gluten-free. This is how to prepare it:

Components:

Regarding Cake:
  Two big oranges
  Six big eggs
  1 cup of sugar, granulated
  two and a third cups of ground almond meal
  A smidgeon of baking powder

Regarding Syrup:
  Two oranges juiced

1/2 cup of sugar, granulated

Guidelines:

Get the oranges ready:
   I begin by giving the oranges a good wash and putting them in a pot. I pour water over them and bring them to a boil. After that, I turn down the heat and simmer them for about two hours. This process eliminates the bitterness and softens the oranges.

Incorporate the oranges:
   I drain the oranges and allow them to cool once they are soft. I then chop them into quarters, take out the seeds, and puree the oranges until they are smooth and pulpy. This puree serves as the cake's colorful foundation.

Warm up the oven:
   I grease an 8-inch round cake pan and preheat the oven to 350°F (175°C). It's similar to laying the groundwork for our zesty invention.

Beat Sugar and Eggs Together:
   I combine the eggs and sugar in a mixing bowl and whisk them until they are pale and foamy, resembling the first notes of a cheery tune.

Mix in the baking powder and almonds:
   I mix in the baking powder and ground almonds (almond meal) very gently. This concoction is comparable to the tastefully chosen instruments in a symphony.

Stir in the Orange Puree.
   I blend the smooth orange puree into the batter by folding it

in. A zesty note is added by the orange puree.

Bake until done:

I fill the cake pan with batter, then pop it into the oven to preheat. A toothpick inserted into the center of the cake should come out clean after 45 to 50 minutes of baking. It is similar to the cake's spectacular display.

Get the orange syrup ready by:

I make the orange syrup while the cake bakes. I put sugar and the juice of two oranges in a saucepan. I simmer it until the syrup thickens and the sugar dissolves. This syrup will give the cake a glaze that is both sweet and zesty.

Allow to Soak:

I pierce the top of the cake several times with a toothpick or skewer after it has come out of the oven. I then cover the cake with the warm orange syrup, letting it seep in and give it a hint of citrus sweetness.

Set and Cool:

I waited for the Orange and Almond Cake to cool in the pan so that it could solidify and take on all the flavors, much like a piece of music approaching its last, harmonious notes.

Present with vigor:

I top the orange zest on the Orange and Almond Cake before serving it. A delightful symphony of citrus and nutty notes, each bite of this gluten-free masterpiece is guaranteed to make your day.

This cake embodies the essence of citrus and almonds, and is more than just a dessert—it's a culinary composition, a symphony of flavors and textures. Savor this wonderful creation!

Fruitful Delights

Poached Pears in Red Wine

Preparing Poached Pears in Red Wine is similar to creating an elegant dessert that is both aesthetically pleasing and delectable. Here's how I make this classy dessert.

Components:
Four ripe but firm pears—Bosc or Anjou are good options—
One bottle of fine red wine, such as Merlot or Cabernet Sauvignon
1 cup of sugar, granulated
two sticks of cinnamon
Four cloves
One orange's zest
Orange juice from one
One split vanilla bean along its length
Vanilla ice cream or whipped cream (optional) for serving

Guidelines:

After peeling, core the pears.

I start by peeling the pears, trying to keep the stems intact. Next, I carefully remove the cores from the bottom using a melon baller or a small spoon, leaving a tiny opening for the wine and spices. The pears take on the appearance of fragile, empty vessels that are ready to hold flavor.

Get the Poaching Liquid ready:

I pour the entire bottle of red wine into a big saucepan. The pears can plunge into it like they are in a rich, deep pool. I add the orange zest, juice, cloves, cinnamon sticks, and granulated sugar, and I stir everything together very gently. This drink, with its zesty citrus notes and warm, spicy undertones, is the essence of our dessert.

Let the Pears Soak:

I make sure the pears are completely submerged in the red wine mixture before adding them. The pears appear to be enjoying a sumptuous soak in the aromatic liquid.

Add the bean of vanilla:

I allow the aromatic vanilla bean to infuse the poaching liquid by adding the split bean to it. It enhances the composition's depth like a faint melody.

Melt Slowly:

I cover the saucepan and bring the poaching liquid to a gentle simmer. Simmer the pears for 25 to 30 minutes, or until they are soft and the wine gives them a rich, ruby-red color. It has a calming, slow rhythm to it.

Take the Pears Out:

I carefully remove the pears from the liquid and transfer them to a serving dish using a slotted spoon. It's like giving our dessert stars a stage of their own.

Cut Down on the Liquid

I simmer the mixture until it thickens and takes on the texture of a rich syrup, akin to a musical crescendo. Our final touch is this syrup.

Accompany with Panache:

I cover the pears with the red wine syrup, giving them a glossy shine. I might serve them with a scoop of vanilla ice cream or a dollop of whipped cream to give them an extra luxurious touch. It's similar to the last note of harmony in our recipe.

Savoring a symphony of flavors with every bite of these Poached Pears in Red Wine is akin to experiencing the warmth of the spices, the sweet elegance of the pears, and the bold, fruity notes of the wine. This dessert is more than just food; it's an encounter. Have fun!

Yogurt with fresh figs and honey

Making Fresh Fig and Honey Yogurt is like creating a simple yet elegant melody of flavors, with the golden touch of honey and the creamy richness of yogurt balancing the natural sweetness of ripe figs. Here's how to make this tasty treat differently:

Components:
Ripe and plump fresh figs with your favorite yogurt variety or Greek yogurt
Raw honey, ideally from nearby
A small amount of toasted nuts, like walnuts or almonds, for crunch (optional)
Garnish with fresh mint leaves (optional).

Guidelines:

Choose the Ideal Figs:
I begin by selecting fresh figs that are plump and ripe. They ought to smell sweet and feel velvety to the touch. Every fig is like a different note in our recipe.

Get the figs ready:
I handle the figs with gentle care, scrubbing and drying them like priceless musical instruments. Next, I trim the stems and cut the figs in half or quarters, depending on how big they are.

Spread the Yogurt Out:
I put a heaping spoonful of Greek yogurt in each bowl or on a serving dish. Yogurt serves as a smooth and mild base note, providing a creamy foundation.

Organize the Slices of Fig:

I layer the sliced figs over the yogurt like how I would arrange notes on a staff. The figs add bright color and natural sweetness in bursts.

Pour some honey on it:
I pour honey over the yogurt and figs, letting it trickle down like a golden, syrupy song. The dish is enhanced by the honey's rich, sweet harmony.

Add the optional toasted nuts:
I top the figs with a handful of toasted nuts, like walnuts or almonds, to add even more flavor and texture. It adds a delightful crunch, akin to the crescendo of a beautiful piece.

Fresh mint is an optional garnish.

I add a few sprigs of fresh mint leaves to the dish if I have any on hand. The mint leaves add a touch of freshness and are like the final touches to our meal.

Handle with elegance:
I present the Yogurt with Fresh Figs and Honey with style and simplicity. A harmonious melody of creamy, sweet, and nutty notes dances on the palate with every bite.

This delicious treat is more than just a snack; it's a gastronomic composition that highlights the beauty of simplicity with a symphony of flavors and textures. Savor the Sweet Experience of Honey and Fresh Fig Yogurt!

Chapter 10: Meal Planning and Tips

This is a 4-week Mediterranean meal plan that is well-balanced. Fruits, vegetables, whole grains, lean meats, and healthy fats are abundant in this diet. In addition to being tasty, it also supports general well-being and heart health.

Week 1:

Day 1:
Breakfast: Greek yogurt with honey and fresh berries.
Lunch: Mediterranean quinoa salad.
Dinner: Grilled chicken with lemon and oregano, a side of roasted vegetables.

Day 2:

Breakfast: Whole grain toast with avocado and tomato.

Lunch: Hummus and veggie wrap.

Dinner: Baked salmon with a side of quinoa and steamed broccoli.

Day 3:

Breakfast: Oatmeal topped with nuts, dried fruits, and a drizzle of honey.

Lunch: Mediterranean chickpea salad.

Dinner: Shrimp and vegetable stir-fry with brown rice.

Day 4:

Breakfast: Scrambled eggs with spinach and feta cheese.

Lunch: Caprese salad with mozzarella, tomatoes, and basil.

Dinner: Baked cod with a side of mixed greens and balsamic vinaigrette.

Day 5:

Breakfast: Whole grain cereal with fresh fruit and Greek yogurt.

Lunch: Greek salad with olives and feta cheese.

Dinner: Grilled eggplant and zucchini with couscous.

Day 6:

Breakfast: Smoothie with spinach, banana, Greek

yogurt, and a drizzle of honey.

Lunch: Lentil soup and a side of mixed greens.

Dinner: Roasted chicken with Mediterranean herb seasoning and a side of brown rice.

Day 7:

Breakfast: Whole grain toast with almond butter and sliced strawberries.

Lunch: Tuna salad with olives and mixed greens.

Dinner: Vegetable and chickpea stew.

Weeks 2-4: You can either experiment with different Mediterranean diet recipes, such as stuffed grape leaves, tabbouleh, or ratatouille, or you can stick to the meals from Week 1. The secret is to emphasize whole, fresh foods and to load your meals with an abundance of fruits, vegetables, nuts, and olive oil.

Drink plenty of water to stay hydrated, and feel free to occasionally sip on a glass of red wine. Additionally, remember to eat with awareness, control your portions, and enjoy the flavors of every meal.

This four-week meal plan follows the Mediterranean diet's tenets while offering a range of flavors and nutrients. Cheers to starting a healthier and more delicious lifestyle!

Building Balanced Mediterranean Meals

Creating well-balanced Mediterranean meals involves not only what you eat but also how you prepare it. It's a way of life that places a focus on eating mindfully and on whole, fresh foods. The following advice will help you prepare first-person, well-balanced Mediterranean meals:

1. Start with Fresh Vegetables: I always serve a variety of fresh vegetables as the first course in my Mediterranean meals. They supply vital vitamins, minerals, and fiber and serve as the plate's base. I try to incorporate a variety of colors into my dishes, such as leafy greens, tomatoes, cucumbers, and bell peppers, which not only add color but also nutrients.

2. Use Whole Grains: Mediterranean cooking uses a lot of whole grains. I adore offering choices like bulgur, brown rice, quinoa, and whole wheat pasta. These grains go well with veggies and proteins because they have a hearty texture and provide sustained energy.

3. Incorporate Lean Proteins: I look to lean foods like poultry, fish, legumes, and nuts for my protein needs. Good sources of omega-3 fatty acids include mackerel, sardines, and salmon. Excellent plant-based options include lentils, beans, and chickpeas. Roasted or grilled lean poultry, such as turkey or chicken, makes a tasty side dish.

4. Embrace Healthy Fats: I use a lot of olive oil in my Mediterranean meals, which is a great source of healthy fats. It

adds a wonderful depth of flavor and is an essential part of the diet. I also like to add nuts, seeds, and avocados to my meals to up the heart-healthy fat content.

5. Add Fresh Herbs and Spices: To improve flavor, add fresh herbs like basil, parsley, and mint along with spices like cumin, thyme, and oregano. Frequently, I use them to season food instead of using a lot of salt.

6. Enjoy Dairy in Moderation: Greek yogurt or small amounts of cheese are my preferred forms of dairy consumption, even though dairy is a staple of the Mediterranean diet. They supply probiotics and calcium without going overboard with saturated fats.

7. Incorporate Fruits Frequently: Ripe oranges, apples, and grapes are a delightful way to cap off a Mediterranean dinner. They provide natural sugars for a hint of sweetness and function as a healthful dessert.

8. Exercise Portion Control: I watch how much I eat to make sure I'm not overindulging. Mediterranean cuisine emphasizes flavor over quantity in dishes.

9. Savor Every Bite: Eating a Mediterranean diet emphasizes eating both what and how you eat. I enjoy the flavors and textures of each bite, taking my time to fully appreciate them. This mindful eating strategy reduces overeating and aids in digestion.

10. Drink Plenty of Water: During Mediterranean meals, water

is the recommended beverage. Throughout the meal, I keep a glass of water on the table and sip from it. I might occasionally enjoy a glass of red wine, but never more than I need.

Creating well-balanced Mediterranean meals is a lifestyle that supports health and happiness, not just a dietary decision. I can make tasty, wholesome meals that are satisfying and beneficial to my general health by using these tips.

Mindful Eating and Portion Control

Maintaining a healthy and balanced diet requires practicing portion control and mindful eating. The following explains each of the two ideas:

Portion control is the art of controlling how much food you consume in a single meal. It makes it easier for you to control how many calories you eat and helps prevent overeating. How to exercise portion control is as follows:

Recognize Serving Sizes: Learn the typical serving sizes for the various food groups. Dietary guidelines or nutrition labels will contain information on this. Understanding what constitutes a "serving" is the first step.

Utilize Measuring Tools: You can measure your food more precisely by using portion control plates, food scales, and measuring cups. This is especially helpful the first few times you learn about portion sizes.

Take Note of Your Body: Observe the signals your body sends when it is hungry or full. You should stop eating even if there is food left on your plate when you are comfortably full.

Don't Eat Straight Out of Packages: When you eat from a big container of ice cream or a bag of chips, it's simple to lose track of how much you've eaten. Instead, divide an appropriate serving into a different dish.

Plate Carefully: Use smaller bowls and plates to present your food. Your mind can be tricked into thinking you can be satisfied with less food if you visually perceive a full plate.

When dining out, share since restaurant servings are frequently bigger than what you require. To save half the meal, think about splitting a dish with your dining partner or promptly requesting a take-out box.

Avoid Super-Sizing: When offered the choice, resist the urge to upgrade to a larger portion. Even if a standard size seems like a better option, stick with it.

The three main components of mindful eating are being present during a meal, savoring every sensory aspect of it, and paying attention to your body's signals. The following is a guide to mindful eating:

Eat Without Distractions: Put your phone away, turn off the TV, and take a seat at a table to eat. Eating while working or in front of a computer can encourage mindless overeating.

Involve Your Senses: Savor the tastes, textures, and scents of your food as you eat. Take note of the hues and arrangement of your dish. The meal is more fully appreciated as a result of this sensory experience.

Chew Slowly: Give your food a good, long chew. It facilitates digestion and enables your brain to recognize fullness.

Savor Every Bite: Let the flavors settle in between bites, then put down your fork. Consider the components and how well they work together.

Assess Your Level of Hunger: Take a moment during your meal to determine how hungry you are. Consider whether you're eating because of habit or boredom or whether you're still hungry.

Show Gratitude: Think about the source of your food and the work that went into making it. This may help you develop a stronger bond with your food.

When you feel satisfied, stop and pay attention to your body's signals. You should stop eating even if there is food left on your plate when you are comfortably full.

You can improve your digestion, avoid overindulging, and create a healthier relationship with food by practicing portion control and mindful eating. Meals that combine these approaches can be more satisfying and well-balanced.

Incorporating Exercise into Your Lifestyle

Including exercise in your daily routine is essential for preserving both your physical and emotional health. It's important to find activities you enjoy and incorporate them into your routine regularly, rather than just going to the gym. Here's how to do it and a selection of various exercise kinds to think about:

1. Pick Pleasurable Activities:

The first step is to choose things that you enjoy doing. Engaging in physical activities you enjoy, such as dancing, hiking, swimming, or sports, can help you maintain an exercise regimen.

2. Make sensible objectives:

Set attainable objectives first, like working out for 30 minutes three times a week. As you get more comfortable, gradually increase the duration and frequency.

3. Plan Out Your Exercise:

Exercise should be regarded as a serious appointment. Make sure to schedule a specific time on your calendar for your workouts, and stick to it every day.

4. Locate a Training Partner:

It can be enjoyable and motivating to work out with a friend. You can support and hold one another responsible for one another.

5. Contrast It:

To keep things interesting and work for different muscle groups, variety is essential. Combine strength training, flexibility training, and cardiovascular exercises.

Kinds Of Workouts

Workouts for the Heart:

These cardiovascular exercises raise your heart rate and strengthen your heart. Choices consist of:

Jogging, running, or walking
cyclizing
Diving and Swimming
Rope jumping exercises

Strength Exercise:

Strength training raises metabolism and results in muscle growth. Weights or bodyweight exercises can be used as resistance. Choices consist of:

Lifting weights
Bodyweight workouts (planks, squats, and push-ups)
Bands of resistance

Yoga (which improves flexibility as well)

Exercises for Flexibility and Balance:

These exercises assist with posture, balance, and flexibility. Choices consist of:
Asana Pilates
Tai Chi Exercises for Stretching

HIIT, or high-intensity interval training:
HIIT entails brief intervals of high-intensity training interspersed with brief rest intervals. It's a productive technique to increase endurance and burn calories.

Recreation and Sports:
Playing sports like basketball, tennis, or soccer can be an enjoyable way to stay active and have a competitive element.

Outdoor Pursuits:
You can stay active and establish a connection with nature by going on hikes, kayaking trips, or trail running.

Group Exercise Programs:
Participating in online or live group fitness classes can offer structure and motivation. Exercises like boot camp, Zumba, and spinning may be taught in classes.

Body-Mind Exercises:
Mind-body practices, such as tai chi and meditation, improve physical flexibility and foster mental and emotional well-being.

Keep in mind that consistency is the most crucial element of exercise in your lifestyle. Getting regular exercise that you enjoy is preferable to shoving yourself into a routine that you detest. You'll eventually reap the mental and physical rewards of leading an active lifestyle.

<h1 style="text-align:center">Summary</h1>

Accept a Mediterranean Way of Life

A dopting a holistic approach to health, well-being, and day-to-day living is what it means to embrace the Mediterranean lifestyle, which extends beyond merely sticking to a diet. The ideal method to adopt a Mediterranean lifestyle is as follows:

1. Appreciate Seasonal and Fresh Foods:
Give fresh, complete foods like vegetables, fruits, whole grains, and lean proteins priority. Whenever possible, use ingredients that are in season and locally sourced. Savor these foods' vivid flavors and hues.

2. Use Olive Oil as Your Primary Fat:
Make extra virgin olive oil your main fat source. In addition

to being heart-healthy, it gives your food a deep, earthy flavor.

3. Frequently Indulge in Seafood:

Make sure to include fish in your meals, especially fatty varieties such as sardines, mackerel, and salmon. They are abundant in heart-healthy omega-3 fatty acids.

4. Accept Nuts and Legumes:

Include legumes in your diet, such as beans, lentils, and chickpeas. These offer fiber and plant-based protein. Nuts provide a satisfying crunch and healthy fats. Have a snack.

5. New Spices and Herbs:

Put a lot of fresh herbs and spices in your food. Mint, thyme, basil, and oregano offer layers of flavor without being overly salty.

6. Complete Grain:

Refined grains should be avoided in favor of whole grains like quinoa, brown rice, and whole wheat bread. They are nutrient and fiber-rich.

7. Consume Cheese in Moderation:

Dairy is allowed in the Mediterranean diet, but only in small amounts. Small portions of cheese and Greek yogurt are popular options.

Keep Hydrated:

The main libation of the Mediterranean diet is water. It is necessary for general health. Enjoy a moderate glass of red wine once in a while because it's high in antioxidants.

9. Make Mindful Food Choices:
Enjoy your food by eating with awareness. In addition to paying attention to the tastes and textures of your food, pay attention to your body's signals of hunger and fullness.

10. Savor Dining with Others: Eat meals with your loved ones and friends. A treasured feature of the Mediterranean way of life is social dining. It improves relationships and makes eating more enjoyable.

11. Take Part in Regular Exercise: - Include regular exercise in your schedule, such as yoga, swimming, or walking. A key component of the Mediterranean lifestyle is physical activity.

12. Make Stress Management a Priority: A well-rounded lifestyle requires stress-reduction practices like mindfulness and meditation. Stress reduction enhances mental health.

13. Get Enough Sleep: Getting enough sleep is essential for good health. Aim for seven to nine hours of sound sleep every night.

14. Spend Time Outside: - Make the most of the Mediterranean's climate by getting outside and exploring the natural world. Simply take in the beauty of nature, go for a stroll by the sea, or go hiking in the mountains.

15. Develop Gratitude: - Show gratitude by enjoying life's small pleasures, such as a tasty dinner, a stunning sunset, or the companionship of close ones.

16. Slow Down: Adopt a more leisurely lifestyle. Give yourself permission to enjoy life and treasure the important times.

17. Never Stop Learning: - Gain as much knowledge as you can about the customs, way of life, and advantages of the Mediterranean diet. Lifelong learning is a journey.

By following these guidelines, you'll experience an increased sense of fulfillment, connection, and well-being in your daily life in addition to the health benefits of the Mediterranean lifestyle. It's an approach to life that encourages harmony and balance.

Your Path to a Heart-Healthy Lifestyle

Starting a journey toward a heart-healthy lifestyle is a deeply personal and life-changing event. Here's my first-hand account of my journey toward heart-healthy living:

1. Realizing Change Is Needed:
   I realized I needed to change my lifestyle, and that was the beginning of my journey. I thought about my eating patterns, exercise routines (or lack thereof), and general health. I realized that maintaining heart health is essential to overall well-being and longevity.

2. Self-Education:
   I prepared myself for the journey ahead by learning about heart health. To learn about the risk factors and heart disease

prevention strategies, I conducted extensive research, read articles, and spoke with medical experts.

3. Adopting a Mediterranean Diet:

I consciously decided to switch to a Mediterranean diet. It required more than just adhering to rules; it required a change in how I felt about food. I started to enjoy the tastes of whole grains, lean meats, olive oil, and fresh vegetables. I enthusiastically welcomed the culinary journey.

4. Prioritizing Exercise:

I made exercise a part of my everyday schedule. It was now a source of delight rather than a chore. Exercise became a vital part of my life, whether it was swimming in the evenings, brisk walks in the morning, or vigorous yoga sessions.

5. Intense Mindfulness Training:

I discovered how crucial mindfulness is for lowering stress, which has been linked to cardiac problems. I found that practicing mindfulness and meditation helped me remain composed and grounded when faced with obstacles in life.

6. Encircling Myself with Help:

I came to see that I couldn't go on this adventure by myself. I turned to my family and friends for support, and they inspired and encouraged me. The experience was enhanced by spending time with loved ones over meals and activities.

7. Frequent Examinations:

Getting regular checkups with the doctor became an essential part of my journey. It was crucial to keep an eye on vital health indicators like cholesterol and blood pressure to monitor my progress and make the required corrections.

8. Creating Practical Objectives:
   To keep my journey manageable and sustainable, I set realistic goals and benchmarks. It was about not going for quick fixes but about making small, long-lasting changes.

9. Highlighting Minor Wins:
   I relished each little accomplishment along the road. Every well-prepared meal, every exercise session, and every encouraging medical report strengthened my resolve to lead a heart-healthy lifestyle.

10. Accepting a Lifelong Adventure: I'm still on my path to living a heart-healthy lifestyle. It's a way of life rather than a destination. To keep my heart at the core of my well-being, I must always be learning, growing, and changing.

My path to living a heart-healthy lifestyle has enhanced my life in many ways in addition to my physical well-being. It is a path of self-nurturing, self-exploration, and profound gratitude for the boon of a sound heart.

Relishing The Journey Towards Heart Health

We've set out on an incredible culinary adventure with "Delicious Mediterranean Delights: Easy Recipes for Beginners to Embrace the Heart-Healthy Lifestyle." We have examined the Mediterranean diet's bright flavors, illustrious history, and healthful goodness.

When we wrap up this culinary journey, keep in mind that it's more than just a collection of recipes—rather, it's a guide to a happier, healthier life. The art of savoring food, life, and every moment is celebrated in the heart-healthy Mediterranean lifestyle. It's a dedication to caring for our souls as well as our bodies.

Fresh veggies, sweet fruits, lean meats, and comforting grains are all abundant in the Mediterranean diet, which has been around for ages. Eating is a symphony of sensory experiences, and the dining table is a place of joy and connection. It is the epitome of balance and mindfulness.

As you go, think of these recipes as a blank canvas on which you can paint your ideas, your tastes, and your passion for healthy living. Make these recipes your own by adding your vibrant touches, and use your kitchen as the canvas on which to paint the culinary portrait of your heart-healthy journey.

We are not alone in our quest to adopt a Mediterranean lifestyle. Meals are communal experiences that are shared around the table with friends and family, giving people the chance to deepen their relationships and make enduring memories.

You've armed yourself with the information, the tastes, and the motivation to keep going in this exploration. Let the heart-healthy values of mindfulness, gratitude, and a slower, more meaningful pace permeate your life as you enjoy the flavors of the Mediterranean.

Your heart deserves to be in tune with every action you take because it is the conductor of this symphony. Every meal, every bite, every day fully experienced is a note in the exquisite composition of a heart-healthy existence.

Thus, carry on with this journey as an ongoing adventure and way of life rather than as a destination reached. a life in which every meal presents an opportunity to embrace happiness, health, and a closer relationship with both the outside world and yourself.

Enjoy every moment, my fellow traveler. The Mediterranean diet is about a lifelong love affair with health, not just recipes.

www.ingramcontent.com/pod-product-compliance
Lightning Source LLC
Chambersburg PA
CBHW050825260726
48660CB00004B/1604